The politics
of
consumer
representation

A study of Community Health Councils

by Rudolf Klein and Janet Lewis

CENTRE FOR STUDIES IN SOCIAL POLICY

Other publications

by the Centre for Studies in Social Policy:

The public expenditure series

Rudolf Klein   *Social Policy and Public Expenditure, 1974* (£1.50 plus postage)

Rudolf Klein (ed.) *Inflation and Priorities, 1975* (£3.50 plus postage)

Quentin Outram   *The Significance of Public Expenditure Plans, 1975* (£2 plus postage)

Rudolf Klein, Martin Buxton and Quentin Outram *Constraints and Choices, 1976* (£2 plus postage)

In addition, there is a series of Centre Working Papers. These include:

English Law and Social Policy

Work and the changing social climate

Notes towards a theory of patient involvement

The distribution of household income in the UK, 1957-1972.

A full list, together with prices, can be obtained on application.

The Bedford Square Press has also published the following on behalf of the Centre:

Tessa Blackstone *Education and day care for young children in need*

Rudolf Klein and Phoebe Hall *Caring for quality in the caring services*

Timothy Raison *The Act and the Partnership*

Michael Fogarty *Forty to Sixty*

Published 1976 by the Centre for Studies in Social Policy
62 Doughty Street, London WC1N 2LS.

ISNB 0 9503317 4 0
© Copyright 1976 Centre for Studies in Social Policy.

Designed and produced by Gemini Publishing, London.
Text set in 11 on 13pt Times New Roman.
Printed by Henry T. Cook & Co. Ltd., London EC1

Contents

Introduction 7

A note about the tables 9

Chapter 1: Inventing an institution 11

Chapter 2: A profile of the members 27

Chapter 3: Views and verdicts 83

Chapter 4: Aspirations, activities
            and frustrations 115

Chapter 5: Policy implications
            and options 151

Appendix A 177

Appendix B — Survey methods 195

Introduction

It is not often that Governments invent new institutions, and so offer an opportunity to study their conception, birth and evolution. When, therefore, the Government set up Community Health Councils in 1974, as part of its reorganisation of the National Health Service, the chance was too good to miss. We decided to look at this institutional experiment from the time of its inception. It seemed interesting for a variety of reasons. Specific to the British NHS, there was the question of whether central accountability and planning could be reconciled with responsiveness to consumer views at the local level, and whether the invention of the Community Health Councils had squared this particular circle. Generally, there was the question of whether separating the consumer-representation role from the service-management function, the dominating idea behind the creation of Community Health Councils, could provide a model for more widespread use in public services in Britain and elsewhere.

Initially, and no doubt over-hopefully, we intended this to be an evaluation study. The aim was to provide a balance sheet, as it were, of the successes and failures of the Community Health Councils in England and Wales — always assuming, of course, that it would be feasible to define what was meant by success or failure in this context. In the event, such an exercise has not been possible. The reason for this is partly that the process of setting up and establishing the Community Health Councils took far longer than envisaged in the original time-table drawn up by the Department of Health and Social Security: although the process of setting up CHCs was supposed to start in April 1974, it had still not been completed in all regions a year later. Equally, the agonies of NHS reorganisation turned out to be much more prolonged than had been anticipated. In practice, CHC members took office in a period of administrative disorganisation and financial disorientation. To try to evaluate Community Health Councils on the basis of their experiences in 1974 and 1975 would therefore be a nonsense. At the time of writing, it is clear that the CHCs have not been in existence long enough to provide evidence for any verdict on their utility or otherwise. What is more, we have become convinced that, given the slow pace of institutional evolution, our initial assumptions about the possibility of reaching any firm conclusions on the basis of a three-year study were over-optimistic even if the process of administrative change had not been so slow.

This, then, is an interim report on Community Health Councils. It describes the policy processes which led to their creation (Chapter 1), reports on a national survey of CHCs members (Chapters 2 and 3), analyses their first year activities (Chapter 4) and concludes by examining some of the policy issues and discussing future options (Chapter 5). The intention in all this is to present the evidence in a way which, we hope, will be useful both to those whose main concern is with the British NHS and to those who are interested in the more general issue of consumerism, participation and representation in public services dominated by professional expertise. Above all, we have used the experience of the CHCs to try to clarify the ideas involved. There are few more cloudy concepts than that of "consumer representation", and the brief history of the CHCs is interesting as a study of the problems involved in giving precise meaning to this phrase of rhetorical uplift. Our approach is therefore analytical rather than descriptive. No attempt is made to give a detailed, blow-by-blow account of the evolution of CHCs. But to provide a picture of how specific CHCs work, four case studies are being published as a separate Working Paper.

In collecting the information on which this report is based, we have been helped by a great many people whose kindness we acknowledge gratefully. There were the politicians and civil servants involved in setting up CHCs who talked to us freely, if off-the-record. There were the officials at both the DHSS and the regional authority headquarters who prepared the way for our survey of CHC members. There were the CHC members and secretaries who co-operated by filling in questionnaires and sending us agendas and minutes. Finally there were the members of our Advisory Group who gave us much sensible guidance about ways and means, but who are in no way responsible for what we did.

We must also stress our appreciation of those who helped us in the execution of the project. The survey of CHC members was carried out, on our behalf, by Social Policy Research Ltd.; the computing of the resulting data was done, with great patience, by Alan Joy; the Centre librarian, Susan Johnson, has unfailingly met our many and varied demands. Above all, Elizabeth Worth took care of all the secretarial and administrative chores. Finally, we want to thank the Centre for Studies in Social Policy for providing the resources and the environment which made this project possible.

Rudolf Klein   Janet Lewis

June, 1976   Centre for Studies in Social Policy

A note about the tables

One of the problems of presenting the data from a national survey is that, inevitably, all of it is of some interest to someone but hardly anything is of interest to everyone. To avoid over-cluttering the analysis with tables, we have therefore limited ourselves to including in the main text only those central to the discussion while relegating the rest to an appendix. The tables in the Appendix are distinguished by having the letter A attached to the number.

In the geographical analysis of data, we have included Wales alphabetically among the English health service regions. In doing so, we have sacrificed strict accuracy to simplicity in presentation, and we hope this explanation to our Welsh readers will anticipate their protests. Because of rounding-off, not all the percentages in the tables add up to precisely 100. In each table, N equals the total numbers on which the percentages have been calculated.

1

Inventing
an institution

In trying to trace the origins of institutional innovations, it is always tempting to re-write Genesis: to search, in other words, for evidence of some deliberate design and a clear sense of purpose. In the case of the Community Health Councils, such an approach would be misleading. In this particular instance, the architect was necessity and the builder was expediency. They were invented almost by accident because, when the plans for a reorganised National Health Service were almost complete, all those involved realised that something was missing: an element which could be presented and seen as providing a degree of local democracy, consumer participation or public involvement in the affairs of the NHS. Effectively CHCs were therefore invented to fill a political vacuum, and their subsequent evolution and the uncertainties about their role reflect their improvised beginning.

To understand this process it is necessary to understand also the circumstances which gave birth to the reorganised NHS. Reorganisation was the child of the belief in centralised planning — in the achievement of a fair and rational deployment of resources — which dominated the 'sixties and survived, despite a change of government, into the early 'seventies: the period which saw the development of long-term public expenditure planning and the introduction of new techniques like PAR and programme budgeting in central government[1]. It was this intellectual approach — a curious sort of hybrid between 19th century Fabianism and 20th century managerialism — which had helped to shape the reorganisation of local government: witness the emphasis on corporate planning. And it was this intellectual approach which dominated the approach to health service reorganisation, from the first Green Paper to the final White Paper. This was not the only aim of policy: reorganisation was also seen as an opportunity to achieve two objectives implicit in the creation of the NHS but frustrated by the circumstances in 1946 — the alignment of NHS administrative boundaries with those of local authorities and the amalgamation of the hospital with the primary care and public health sectors. But no account of reorganisation can make sense without taking into account the desire to achieve both greater social equity and a higher degree of efficiency in the use of resources by means of a more effective system of central control.

Equally, and more specific to the NHS, the 'sixties were a period of growing awareness of the failures of the existing system to bring about desired changes. On the one hand, there was the evidence that one of the main objectives in setting up the NHS — the achievement of a more equitable geographical distribution of resources[2] — had not been attained. On the other hand, there was a growing realisation of a persisting imbalance between the resources devoted to different sections of the population: in particular, a series of scandals[3] revealed the financial under-nourishment of the long-stay sector of the NHS. In both cases, the conclusion appeared to be the same once again: that there was a need, first, to use available resources more efficiently and, second, to strengthen the ability of central government to give greater priority to the hitherto neglected areas of the NHS.

The logic of these considerations neatly fitted into the prevailing fashion for centralised planning. As Richard Crossman, a Labour Secretary of State for Social Services, saw it, the need was to destroy the "oligarchies" who had hitherto dominated the Regional Hospital Boards[4] and so perpetuated the historic pattern of health care. As Sir Keith Joseph, a Conservative Secretary of State for Social Services, saw it, the need was to "balance needs and resources rationally" to replace a system where things "just happened" by one in which priorities could be identified and enforced[5]. The language changed as governments and Secretaries of State changed; the basic purpose did not. As one Green Paper succeeded another, some of the institutional expressions of the purpose were modified — in particular the role of the regions and the composition of the authorities. But with the only alternative option to a centralised system, local government control, effectively ruled out by both parties as theoretically desirable but politically impracticable, the scope for ideological variations on the basic theme of policy was limited.

The implications of maintaining a centrally financed NHS, with the Secretary of State responsible to Parliament for the expenditure and the choice of priorities, were reinforced by the emphasis on introducing and implementing change from the centre. It meant that Nye Bevan's phrase about the Regional Hospital Boards being the "agents" of central government, and the Hospital Management Committees being in turn the "agents" of the RHBs, would have to be translated from political rhetoric into administrative reality under the new arrangements. The emphasis on accountability upwards followed inevitably and inescapably: if central control and answerability to Parliament signified anything, it meant that the new Regional Health Authorities and Area Health Authorities would have to be accountable hierarchically.

The effect of this change was compounded by a feature special to the Conservative proposals, and fiercely resisted by the Labour Party. This was the insistence that the members of the new authorities would be chosen for their personal qualities, and not as representatives of either the local authorities or of the professions working in the NHS. The logic of this decision was impeccable: upward accountability is scarcely compatible with accountability to local communities or professional peers (and if representative members were not so answerable, then what was representative about them?). But the political consequences were distinctly uncomfortable. It meant that, following the massacre of HMC members which at a stroke removed the largest element of lay participation in the management of the NHS, there was a conspicuous absence of anything remotely resembling consumer representation in the reorganised service. And although the plans for reorganisation had begun to evolve in the mid'sixties, the era of interest in planning, they had been completed in the 'seventies, the era of interest in participation. The political problem, therefore, was how to best square the circle of élitism and populism: how to reconcile the emphasis on centralised planning with the currently fashionable rhetoric of local participation.

The answer was to invent the Community Health Councils: to add, as it were, a Gothic Folly to the Palladian Mansion — but to do so in a way which would not destroy the basic symmetry (as much intellectual as architectural) of the main building. "The idea suggested itself", in the words of one of the Ministers involved, "as soon as we had decided to go for unrepresentative AHAs". As the participants saw it, CHCs were thus the necessary response to the political challenge of reconciling "the emphasis on mangerial efficiency and non-representative authorities with the fact that a representative element had been promised by Richard

Crossman". Moreover, CHCs also appeared to fill another, more positive function: that of encouraging co-operation between the health and personal social services — a strong personal commitment of Sir Keith Joseph, the Secretary of State — by involving the local community in the NHS. Indeed some of the early discussions about the CHCs took place at the DHSS in the context of meetings not about consumer representation but about how best to integrate services at the local level.

Some sort of representative body at the district level had, of course, already been outlined in the 1970 Green Paper[6] published by Crossman. This was the district committee made up of "a chairman and half the members appointed by and drawn from the Area Health Authority and the other half drawn from people living or working in the district". Their functions were left somewhat vague: they were to have no separate budget and no statutory powers. But their purpose, in as far as it was stated, was both to supervise the running of services — as the agents of the AHA — and to serve "as one of the channels through which local people can keep the area health authority informed of any problems they encounter with the local health services". In short (to note another stream of administrative expediency which fed into the development of CHCs) district committees as originally conceived seem largely to have been a response not to demands for local participation but to the realisation that most of the Areas would be so large as to compel administrative devolution to districts within them. Having abolished the old HMCs, the 1970 Green Paper resurrected something very much like them in the shape of the new district committees.

The drafters of the Conservative proposals, therefore, faced a double task when it came to devising the CHCs. First, there was the need for political differentiation: presentationally it had to be made clear that CHCs were no relation of the district committee. Second, there was the problem of making the CHCs compatible with the managerial philosophy which informed the over-all design. Fortunately, both considerations pointed in the same direction: the separation of the managerial and the representative functions. The district committee proposals, the 1971 Consultative Document argued, would have led to "a dangerous confusion between management on the one hand and the community's reaction to management on the other". "Public opinion", to quote the subsequent 1972 White Paper, would be given its own platform: instead of confusing the "direction of services and representation", each function was to have its own institutions so as to avoid the blurring of roles.

The theory was persuasive, and there was at least some evidence that in practice the old system of combining the managerial and the critical roles had caused difficulties: the report on conditions at Ely hospital[7] had, for example, underlined the problems of HMC members "in combining the role of 'consumer representation' with that of management", and the findings of the inquiry suggested that many of them were over-dependent on the advice of their officers and inhibited in their defence of the patient interest by a fear of imperilling staff morale. So there was a certain intellectual logic in resolving this dilemma by separating the two roles, which appeared to be pulling in opposite directions. Moreover, many of the arguments against conflating managerial and representative functions had been anticipated even earlier and in a different context: in the 1967 report of the Committee on the Management of Local Government[8] . This recommended that local authorities should be organised in a way not unlike the NHS in terms of the relationship between AHAs and CHCs as it eventually emerged. There would be a small management group of councillors responsible for taking all decisions and supervising the work of the officers: the equivalent of the AHA. And the rest of the councillors would sit on committees which "should not be directing or controlling bodies" but would, among other duties, "consider the interests, reactions and criticisms of the public and convey them to the officers and if necessary to the management board": the equivalent of the CHC. Significantly, perhaps, while the Maud model helps to explain some of the intellectual antecedents of NHS reorganisation, it was in practice rejected by local authorities.

Opinion within the DHSS was not, in any case, unanimous about the wisdom of setting up CHCs as independent, non-executive bodies. In the discussions at the department, in as far as they can be reconstructed from the memories of participants, there were some who were worried lest the CHCs — deprived of all direct responsibilities — would become "naggers and stirrers up of complaints". Others simply thought that the CHCs would be ineffective. No systematic attempt appears to have been made to look at the experience of the consultative machinery in the nationalised industries; everyone concerned is clear that these did not provide lessons, far less a model, for CHCs. In short, once the basic idea had been accepted, the composition and functions of CHCs were extemporised rather than being derived either from a precise blue-print or from a model: "We first decided that there should be such a body and then decided what it should do. As we worked on the CHCs, we found more things for them to do".

It is therefore not surprising that the sections of the NHS reorganisation

Bill dealing with the CHCs provide, on the face of it, interesting case-material in support of the thesis that parliamentary opinion can still affect legislation. A number of significant changes were made in response to backbench prodding in the Lords and Commons[9] . Initially the proposal was that half the CHCs members were to be appointed by local authorities and half by AHAs; under pressure (from the Government's own supporters as well as the opposition), the composition was changed to be half nominated by local authorities, one-third chosen by voluntary organisations and one sixth selected by the Regional Health Authorities. Again, responsibility for financing and accommodating CHCs was transferred from the AHAs to the RHAs. The idea of a national organisation for CHCs[10] was introduced into the Bill, which allowed, though it did not bind, the Secretary of State to set up such a body. Unfortunately for those who believe that the influence of Parliament can be measured by the number of amendments made by backbenchers to Government legislation[11] , the reason why Ministers were prepared to change the original Bill was that CHCs were peripheral to the main architecture of the new NHS. Ministers, to quote one of them, had "no fixed ideas about how they should be constituted or how they should work. We were much happier to make concessions on this part of the Bill than on the management structure. And it always helps politically to able to make some concessions". In other words, the apparent influence of Parliament may — the case of the CHCs would suggest — simply reflect lack of ministerial and departmental certainty.

But while CHCs may have started out as a symbolic nod in the general direction of democracy and participation, their development suggests that symbolic substitutes for action may paradoxically turn into a practical commitment to action. "We were forced to take an interest in them", one of those involved in the process of developing the institution recalls, "because of the interest taken in them". And it is precisely the gap between any precise definition of their role and purpose in the first place and the practical administrative necessity of giving shape and form to them which helps to explain some of the basic ambiguities about what they should actually do — the source of many of the problems discussed in a subsequent chapter, which deals with the experience of the CHCs in the first year of their existence.

One of the central ambiguities emerges clearly when the phrases used to describe their role are analysed in detail. Ministers and civil servants are not accustomed to read works of political theory as light relief at bed-time, and there is perhaps no reason why they should. But confusion about theory — or, to put it less pompously, lack of clarity about the meaning of words in common use in the political vocabulary — can cause practical problems. Thus every Ministerial speech and every DHSS document implied that the CHCs would have some sort of representative role. But equally almost every speech and document implied different concepts of representation.

The ambiguity emerges clearly when some of the phrases used to define the role of CHCs are compared. Thus the 1972 White Paper described CHCs as "bodies to represent the views of the consumer", which would be made up of "people with particular interest in health services". But, introducing the second reading debate, Lord Aberdare[12] stated that "their basic function will be to represent the interests of the public in each health district". To point to the difference may seem like a pedantic quibble about words; in fact the practical implications of the two definitions are considerable. For the interests of NHS consumers are not necessarily identical with the interests of the local community as a whole; equally to define the constituency of CHCs as the *users* of health services is different from defining it as including non-users. The practical importance of this distinction emerged in the implementation stage of introducing CHCs: when it came to the choice of voluntary organisations eligible to nominate CHC members, there was some confusion (and some difference of policy as between the various RHAs) about whether all organisations should be eligible or only those with a specific health service interest.[13]

There are, of course, further problems about giving specific meaning to the concept of representation, and it is worth teasing these out in some detail since any assessment of the actual composition of CHCs (see below) depends on the initial assumptions made. One such concept, frequently held but seldom explicitly justified, is the "mirror of the community" view of representation[14]. This is usually taken to mean that the composition of representative bodies should reflect the composition of the community.

But what are the relevant measuring-rods for analysing and comparing the composition of the community and the composition of representative bodies? Conventionally, in studies of representatives like local authority members[15], it is assumed that the relevant characteristics are social class, education and demographic factors like age. In our survey of CHC members we have accordingly classified them in these ways. This has the obvious utility of being able to compare CHC membership with the membership of other public bodies. However, there are very severe limitations about the usefulness of this approach — which, as it were, treats representative bodies as though they were the permanent sample in an on-going public opinion poll and concludes that they must accordingly be designed to be an accurate reflection of the population being surveyed. It is to assume that those chosen because they are, say, unskilled workers, educated at elementary schools only and aged over 65 are representative of all unskilled workers, educated at elementary schools and aged over 65. This is more than doubtful. First, the very fact that people are prepared to put themselves forward for selection — and ready to give up time — suggests that they may be unrepresentative: it indicates (a point which will be developed in the analysis of our survey results) that they may already be atypical in being part of the network from which public persons are recruited. Further, if it is assumed that representation implies voicing the values, attitudes and experience of those being represented, it does not follow that the heterogeneity of these can be captured in social class or demographic categories: for instance, the values, attitudes and experience of an agricultural labourer may differ greatly from those of a mineworker (which is of course why public opinion surveys use very much bigger samples than those offered by public bodies of 30 members, and why approaching the problem of representation as though it were an exercise in designing a sample for market research is less than helpful).

The difficulty is not much eased if the relevant community is defined to be the users of the NHS rather than the population at large. Rather it is aggravated. For in addition to the difficulties already discussed, there is the further complication of deciding whether representation ought to be weighted to reflect the intensiveness of use. Health services are used disproportionately by families with young children and the elderly, for example [16]. If the universe of the CHCs were defined as the consumers of the NHS — rather than the community at large — then to be representative, on the "mirror" principle at any rate, they would therefore have to contain a disproportionately high number of pregnant women and pensioners.

There is, however, a different way of looking at representation. This is to view the community not in terms of the characteristics of the individuals composing it, but of the shared interests which these individuals have. This approach puts the emphasis on providing representation for those organised group interests which collect, aggregate and articulate the opinions, wants and preferences of individual citizens. Again, this has its problems. In particular, it raises the question of how to secure representation for those interests which are not organised, or where the members of the groups may be lacking in the confidence, competence or resources (political and financial) required to gain access to the world of policy-making[17] .

In theory, the distinction between these various approaches to the problem of representation may be relatively neat. In practice, the political and administrative decisions about the composition of the CHCs were inevitably taken in a much less tidy and intellectually coherent way. But they do suggest an attempt to hold a balance between representation for the community at large and for special interests among NHS consumers.

In a rough and ready sort of way, the 50% of CHC members nominated by local authorities were seen as representing the community in some undefined way. Additionally, this would have the advantage, it was thought, of encouraging co-operation between local government and the NHS. Furthermore, one of the main themes running through the whole parliamentary debate on reorganisation was the often reiterated belief that the presence of local authority members — whether on CHCs or AHAs would in itself inject an element of democracy into the system. This view was expressed with special force by Labour MPs and peers, although it was not confined to them. And it was the 1974 Labour Government which subsequently increased the number of local authority members on AHAs[18] .

The proposition that the presence of local authority members on NHS bodies can be equated with democracy — "the most promiscuous word in the world of public affairs"[19] — is questionable. It rests on the extremely dubious assumption that the very fact of election is a sort of holy oil of representative legitimacy: that someone elected to serve on one specific body thereby acquires a universal credit card which allows him or her to represent the community in a totally different capacity. But, in practice, this issue was not raised. Putting half the CHC membership into the gift of the local authorities had the advantages of administrative simplicity and political acceptability.

As against these representatives of the community, the third of CHC members chosen by voluntary organisation can be seen as an answer to the problem of ensuring representation for special interests. But it would be a mistake to imply that this was the main motive for involving voluntary organisations in the first place. Just as it was thought desirable to include local authority members in order to encourage co-operation between local government and the NHS, so it was thought desirable to include voluntary organisation members in order to promote their participation in providing support for the NHS. The Conservative Government's policy was, in any case, to encourage voluntary participation in the social services; and,

Richard Crossman's experience at the DHSS had also convinced him of the necessity of promoting this trend[20]. The methods of choosing voluntary organisation members subsequently emerged in response to parliamentary hostility to the idea of selection by AHAs and the need to find some acceptable way of electing them. Once again policy was improvised, largely in a dialogue between the DHSS and the National Council of Social Service, co-ordinating the views of the voluntary organisations.

The solution that emerged was outlined by the National Council in its guidance to local voluntary organisations as to how they might set about choosing their share of CHC members. This suggested that these CHC members should be elected by constituencies, each of whom would represent a particular group of health service users: namely, children, the elderly, the mentally ill or handicapped, the physically handicapped and a general category. Thus, in the event, there was an attempt to bias the selection process in order to ensure representation for the most vulnerable minorities: the criteria used were not numbers but degree of need and lack of political resources.

The role of the DHSS in the setting-up process was recessive. Just as it was left to the National Council for Social Service to orchestrate the selection procedures for voluntary organisations, so it was left to the Regional Health Authorities to decide which of the voluntary organisations should be allowed to take part in the process. Similarly, the RHAs were given only the most general guidance as to the principles to be followed in choosing their sixth of CHC members. The DHSS's circular of advice [21] suggested that, apart from appointing men and women with previous health service experience, their regional sixth should also include "representatives of bodies such as women's organisations, trade-unions, the Churches, the youth and immigrant bodies who might not otherwise be appointed". This, is very much off the Whitehall peg: these are largely the categories which tend, as a matter of routine, to be included on official committees and advisory bodies.

In adopting this strategy the central policy makers appear to have made a virtue of necessity. Since the criteria for selecting CHC members were by no means self-evident — and since there might well be conflicting views as to which interests should be represented, and how, — it suited the DHSS to decentralise the implementation process. In this way, the DHSS was able both to demonstrate its belief in local decision-making and to cushion itself against the inevitable criticisms which would be made by disappointed, would-be members of CHCs. Uncertainty about the aims being pursued and a wish to diffuse blame reinforced the desire of the administrators to devolve the burdens involved in actually setting up CHCs.

One issue about representation was largely ignored, however, although it is central when it comes to assessing the actual composition of CHCs. This is whether those chosen should be representative in their personal characteristics — the "mirror of society" model — or whether they should possess particular skills or competence and thus be unrepresentative of the population as a whole. Taking an extreme case, the answer to this question is fairly self-evident: no one would suggest that the mentally handicapped or the confused elderly should be represented by the mentally handicapped or the confused elderly. But, even leaving this particular example aside, it would be only too easy to imagine a CHC which might be cross-section of the community — in terms of social class, education, age and other similar characteristics — but which might yet be composed of people lacking the competence required to perform the tasks set to them. To assess whether or not the method of selecting CHC members has produced a potentially effective system of representation, therefore means also analysing the tasks set to them — and the kind of qualities implicitly required if they are to be carried out.

The extent to which the role of CHCs had grown, from the original modest conception of voicing the views of the community, became apparent in 1974 when the DHSS published its list of "matters to which Community Health Councils might wish to direct their attention"[22]. These included: the effectiveness of services being provided; the planning of services; collaboration between the health services and local authorities; assessing the extent to which district health facilities conform with the published Departmental policies; the share of available resources devoted to the care of patients unable to protect their own interests, especially those living in hospital for long periods or indefinitely; facilities for patients; waiting periods; quality of catering; and monitoring the volume and type of complaints received about a service or institution.

No one reading this list could complain that the CHCs were being restricted in their activities: it appeared to be an eloquent and effective reply by the Government to those of its critics who argued that the CHCs were too restricted in their role to be effective. But, unfortunately, improvisation also led to difficulties.

Instead of merely being required to collect information from users, actual and potential, CHC members were now being asked to elicit information about the services provided and sit in judgement on the adequacy of the NHS in their district. The list would require the ideal CHC member to spend considerable time mastering the data needed to carry out his or her task of assessing standards, investigating conditions and getting involved in the planning process. Even allowing for the division of labour among CHC members, was this compatible with the methods of selection? Was this designed to produce councillors with the necessary time and skills?

Moreover, as the role of the CHC was expanded, so it appeared to move further away from the original conception. This, as pointed out at the beginning, was to separate management and community representation. But what does management consist of, if not in assessing standards, investigating conditions and getting involved in the planning process? The attempt to square the circle — to give the CHCs a constructive role to play, while yet keeping them out of the management structure of the NHS — turned out, in the event, to be a recipe for friction and misunderstanding: this, indeed, is one of the themes of the chapter which examines the experience of the CHCs during their first year. Policy improvisation was, in this particular instance, also to lead to policy problems.

These problems were further compounded, in the event, by other developments within the reorganised NHS. The neat theoretical antithesis between representative and managerial bodies became increasingly blurred in practice, and was indeed specifically repudiated by the Labour Administration which took office in 1974. Its Consultative Document on Democracy in the National Health Service[23] declared that "The Government do not accept that it is possible or desirable to make such a clear-cut distinction between management of public services and representation of consumer interests and views". Accordingly, the Secretary of State decided both to introduce the idea of elected staff representatives and, as noted above, to increase the number of local authority members on AHAs. The latter, it was hoped, would "provide a link with the people whom they had been elected to represent on the local authority", as well as strengthening co-operation between the NHS and local government. This represented a considerable shift of emphasis from the job-description for AHA members given in the 1972 Grey Book[24]. This sternly reminded AHA members to "focus the limited time of the Authority itself on the critical policy, planning and resource allocation decisions which will shape services to be provided to the people of the Area" and to "ensure that progress is according to agreed objectives, targets and budgets and that services are being provided with efficiency and economy".

At the same time, the Labour Government was anxious to "strengthen the role" of CHCs. It therefore introduced a number of changes. For example, CHCs were encouraged to recruit their secretaries by open competition instead of giving priority to existing members of the NHS staff. And, perhaps more important, it was decided that, given agreement by the CHC, it would no longer be necessary to seek the approval of the Secretary of State for the closure of hospitals. Thus NHS authorities were given a direct incentive to consult CHCs about hospital closures — always a contentious issue, likely to stir up local passions — in order to avoid the long delays involved in seeking DHSS sanction. But (an echo of earlier fears about the danger of CHCs adopting a negatively obstructionist attitude) Community Health Councils which did object to closures were expected "to make a detailed and constructive counter-proposal, with full regard for the factors, including restraints on resources, which have led the health authority to propose the closure". Once again, therefore, CHCs were given a quasi-managerial role to play — just as the AHAs were given a quasi-representative function. Indeed the blurring of roles would have been more pronounced still if the Government had persisted with its tentative proposal for allowing CHCs to elect some of the AHA members as outlined in the Consultative Document — which even raised the possibility of permitting concurrent membership of CHCs and AHAs.

Overall, the evidence discussed would suggest that it would be a mistake to try to assess the record of the CHCs so far exclusively in terms of the intentions of the policy makers who set them up — even assuming that CHCs have been in existence long enough to make such an attempt worthwhile. These intentions were never clear-cut and precise enough to allow them to be tested against experience. The aim of the following chapters will, therefore, be to examine the effects of the policy decisions taken — some predictable, some unexpected — and to look at the problems created by the expectations generated as a result of this experiment in inventing a new institution to fill a political vacuum.

1 Sir Richard Clarke *New Trends in Government* Civil Service College Studies No.1 HMSO 1971.

2 R.F.L. Logan, J.S.A. Ashley, Rudolf Klein and D.M. Robson *Dynamics of Medical Care* Memoir No.14. London School of Hygiene and Tropical Medicine, 1972.

3 Rudolf Klein 'Policy problems and policy perceptions in the National Health Service' *Policy & Politics* Vol.2 No.3. March 1974.

4 R.H.S. Crossman *A politician's view of health services planning*, University of Glasgow 1972.

5 Secretary of State for Social Services *National Health Service Reorganisation: England* HMSO 1972. Cmnd.5005.

6 Department of Health and Social Security *National Health Service: The Future Structure of the National Health Service* HMSO 1970. For an elaboration of the district committee concept, see also the Secretary of State's speech: House of Commons Hansard, Vol.798 No.85, 23 March 1970 cols 1005/6.

7 *Report of the Committee of Inquiry into Allegations of Ill-Treatment of Patients and other irregularities at the Ely Hospital, Cardiff* HMSO 1969, Cmnd.3975. Earlier still, the Guillebaud Committee had also considered this problem and had concluded: "We have no doubt in our own minds that the Health Ministers must reserve to themselves the sole right to decide who shall be appointed to the Regional Boards, and that members must be selected solely for the contribution they can make to the efficient running of the hospital service". However, the Committee also remarked: "The Regional Hospital Boards are intended — at least in part — to represent the community, and in our view, if they were transformed into small bodies of paid 'Directors', their whole character would be changed". *Report of the Committee of Enquiry into the cost of the National Health Service*, HMSO 1956. Cmnd.9663, paras.253/264.

8 Committee on the Management of Local Government (Chairman: John Maud) *Vol.1 Report of the Committee* HMSO 1967.

9 For a detailed account of the changes made during the Bill's passage through Parliament, see David Phillips 'Community Health Councils' in Kathleen Jones (ed.) *The Year Book of Social Policy in Britain, 1974*. Routledge and Kegan Paul 1975.

10 Proposed in Rudolf Klein 'Why health councils need an injection of expertise' *The Times* 26 January 1973. For a discussion of the role of supporting expertise in the context of consumer representation in the nationalised industries, see William A. Robson *Nationalized Industry and Public Ownership* (second edition) Allen & Unwin 1962. See also the evidence of the Public Enterprise Group in Second Report from the Select Committee on Nationalised Industries, Session 1970-1971 *Relations with the public* pp.531-536, HMSO 1971, HC 514.

11 The most laborious example of this sort of analysis is J.A.G. Griffith *Parliamentary Scrutiny of Government Bills* Allen & Unwin 1974.

12 House of Lords Hansard Vol.337, No.16, Col.15. 4 December 1972.

13 For a discussion of the setting-up process, see Rudolf Klein and Janet Lewis 'Community Health Councils — The Early Days' *Health and Social Services Journal* 7 December 1974.

14 Hanna Pitkin *The concept of representation* University of California. Press 1967.

15 For example, see Committee on the Management of Local Government Vol.2 *The Local Government Councillor* HMSO 1967.

16 Office of Population Censuses and Surveys *The General Household Survey, 1973,* HMSO 1976, Section 6.

17 The literature bearing on this point is vast. But, for a selection, see Peter Bachrach and Morton Baratz 'Two faces of power' *American Political Science Review,* December 1962: K. Newton 'A critique of the pluralist model' *Acta Sociologica* Vol.12 No.4 1969; Steven Lukes *Power* Macmillan 1974.

18 Department of Health and Social Security *Democracy in the National Health Service: Membership of Health Authorities* HMSO 1974.

19 Bernard Crick *In Defence of Politics* Penguin 1964.

20 R.H.S. Crossman *The role of the volunteer in the modern social service* Clarendon Press 1973.

21 Department of Health and Social Security *Community Health Councils* HRC (74)4.

22 Ibid, Appendix 5.

23 See note 18, above.

24 Department of Health and Social Security *Management Arrangements for the Reorganised National Health Service* HMSO 1972.

2

A profile
of the members

The characteristics of the men and women who emerge from Britain's political processes to play a representative public role — whether as members of Parliament or as parish councillors — have long attracted interest. There have been a variety of studies [1] which have analysed the composition of representative bodies and which have thrown up a mass of information about the age, education, social class and occupation of various types of representatives. It therefore seems appropriate to start any study of the Community Health Councils with a collective profile of their membership. Here is a new institution designed to promote consumer representation in the National Health Service, with a uniquely eccentric system for choosing the membership. So the most obvious question would seem to be how different CHC members are from representatives chosen by more conventional methods and in other contexts.

This chapter, then, presents the results of a national survey of all CHC members in England and Wales carried out as soon as possible after they took office. It provides a snapshot of the membership at the time of their appointment, but does not attempt to record the effects of the many changes caused by wastage among the original recruits. It examines the characteristics of the members themselves, the extent to which these are linked to the methods of selection and, where possible, the relationship between the composition of the CHCs and that of the communities which they represent.

In sketching this collective profile, we have used the conventional tools of social portraiture. We have analysed the members by age and sex, by social class and education, and so on. This approach has the advantage of using the familiar language of social inquiry, and so permitting a comparison of our results with those of other studies of representative men and women. But it also has the disadvantage of accepting the limitations of this language. This kind of analysis provides information about who people are and what experience they bring to their representative role; it does not tell us how they are likely to view a particular situation or predict how they will react to a specific problem. And indeed we make no attempt to analyse the relationship (if any) between social variables and representative behaviour, though such an exercise might well be worth doing when the CHC's have been in existence long enough to provide a sufficient fund of information about their activities.

Our purpose in analysing the composition of the CHC membership in detail is different. It is to look at the membership in the light of the various theories of representation, discussed in the previous chapter, and to see whether the members thrown up by the system satisfy any of the various and competing criteria by which representative institutions tend to be assessed. The CHCs themselves mirror a political compromise: they are the end-product of the somewhat tortuous process of political bargaining and administrative improvisation described in the previous chapter. To what extent do the CHCs, in turn, reflect the community and in which respects? How far can they claim to represent — in one sense or another of this chameleon word — the consumer interests within the National Health Service?

In trying to answer these questions, our analysis is constrained by the limitations of the data obtained from our national survey (see Appendix B for details of the questionnaire and the response rates) and of that available from other sources. To avoid clumsy circumlocutions, we talk about CHC members throughout this chapter when referring to the respondents of our survey. But, of course, a certain caution is obligatory when equating the CHC membership as a whole with the near-two-thirds of them who actually filled in our questionnaire. While we have no evidence of any systematic pattern of under-representation, neither do we know how different, if at all, the non-responders were from the rest of the survey population. In discussing the national picture, and even when looking at variations between the regions, these statistical considerations are not too inhibiting — though they mean that we tend to disregard small differences in the figures produced by our analysis of the data. But when it comes to discussing differences between individual CHCs, we can only use the evidence illustratively and have made no attempt to present the data for all the CHCs — and have, furthermore, excluded those with a low response rate from even this limited exercise [2] . Given the small numbers on any one CHC — 30 or fewer members — there is always the possibility that information from, say, five non-respondents would have produced a very different picture.

There is a further inhibition on our analysis. The boundaries of the administrative areas of the NHS which are relevant to this inquiry — the regions and the districts — are peculiar to the health service. In attempting to compare the composition of the CHC membership with that of the relevant communities, there is therefore a scarcity of relevant data from the census and other sources. If at times our analysis seems somewhat arbitrary in its selection of factors to compare, it is because the whole exercise has been constrained by the nature of NHS administrative boundaries and the availability of the appropriate information.

The distorting mirror

If representation is defined to mean holding up an accurate mirror to the population being represented, then Community Health Councils are not representative. They do not conform to what might be called the naive theory of representation. In their personal characteristics, the members of CHCs — taken as body — are extremely unrepresentative of the community at large. Only 10% of the total membership are under 35, as against 35% of the population as a whole; there is a middle-aged bulge in the CHC membership, and the over 65s are slightly under-represented (Table 2.1). Over half their members are men, although women are in a majority in the population at large (Table 2.2). More pronouncedly still, they are predominantly middle-class (Table 2.3). They have nearly four times as many members drawn from the professional classes — for example, medical practitioners, judges, university teachers and architects — as the population as a whole: 18% as against 4.9%. They have twice as many members drawn from the intermediate occupations — for instance, nurses, school teachers, managers. shop owners and farmers — as the national total: 36% as against 18% (from this point on, we usually combine these two categories of Social Classes I and II and describe them as "professionals and managers"). They also have far more than their share of Social Class III, i.e. other non-manual workers like clerks, salesmen and draughtsmen: 27% as against 10.2% (from now on referred to, in shorthand terms, as "white-collar workers"). In contrast only 15% of their members are manual workers in Social Classes IV, V and VI — overwhelmingly drawn from the first of the groups, the skilled — while the equivalent figure for the total population is over 58% (subsequently this category carries the label "blue-collar workers"). Particularly striking is the under-representation of working-class women. Only eight per cent of all women members of CHCs come from households headed by blue-collar workers [3].

In all these respects, CHC members show many similarities with public persons in general (Tables 2.1 to 2.3). The available information about local councillors is now almost 10 years out of date, since it was collected for the Committee on the Management of Local Government [4] in the mid-sixties and no similar national survey has been carried out since. Even so the profile of the CHC membership shows a strong family resemblance to that of the councillors in the 'sixties. Both have more in common with each other than either has with the population at large. In each case there is a deficit of the under 35s, although the local councillors in the 'sixties had a relative excess of the over 65s. In each case, too, the middle-classes are heavily over-represented, although the composition of the CHC membership is more heavily weighted with professionals. Although little is known about members of NHS committees, the available evidence [5] suggests that these tend to be even more unrepresentative of the population at large than either CHC or local authority members.

Some of the other characteristics of CHC members follow from the findings already discussed. Given that seven out of ten are over 45, it is not surprising, for example, that (Table 2.4) over four-fifths of them are married and that two-thirds of them have no children under 16. If they represent anyone, it is the solidly established and settled citizen, well-entrenched in his or her own community: two-thirds of CHC members have lived in the district which they represent for more than 15 years, and only one tenth of them have lived there for less than five years. Again, given their social background, it follows that most of them went to a public or grammar school while less than half went to a secondary or elementary school (Table 2.5). Predictably, too, CHC members include a disproportionate number of people who have been to some institution or other of further education: a third have been to a university, a polytechnic or a teacher training college (Table 2.6).

In one respect, however, the CHC members are more representative of the population as a whole than might have been expected: in their employment status (Table 2.7). In contrast to local authority councillors in the 'sixties, the proportion of CHC members working full time and part-time is virtually identical to that in the total population and there is a less pronounced excess of retired people — partly because a surplus of male pensioners is balanced by a deficit of retired women. Interestingly, a tenth of all CHC members — and a fifth of the women among them — work in an unpaid capacity for more than eight hours a week; unfortunately there are no equivalent figures for the population as a whole, so it is impossible to say with certainty whether or not the CHC members are exceptional in this respect.

So far the collective profile of the CHC membership has been based exclusively on national figures. As a result, the picture is something of a caricature. Its bold lines and simple colours exaggerate and distort. On closer inspection, the evidence suggests a more complex, more interesting and more puzzling situation. When the national figures are broken down by regions — and even more, when the regional figures are broken down

Figure 2.1   Regional contrasts

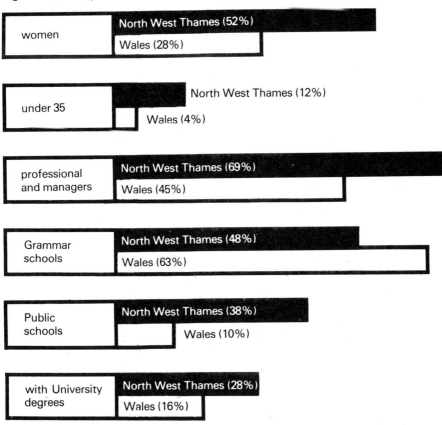

	North West Thames	Wales
women	52%	28%
under 35	12%	4%
professional and managers	69%	45%
Grammar schools	48%	63%
Public schools	38%	10%
with University degrees	28%	16%

by individual councils — it becomes clear that the membership of CHCs, while still in no sense a photoplate image of the community as delineated in census returns, shows a considerable geographical heterogeneity. Nationally, CHC members may be an unrepresentative set of people, in the sense of failing to mirror the population at large. But regionally and locally, the composition of the membership seems to be sensitive to the social and political culture of specific communities [6] . Even though our evidence does not permit us to relate local variations to specific circumstances in particular geographical areas, it does show that the character of the populations being represented does appear to affect the composition of the representatives.

The extent of the regional variations can best be illustrated by looking at some of the extremes (Figure 2.1 and Tables 1A to 5A). The North West Thames region is remarkable for having an above average proportion of CHC members who are women, who are under 35, who are in Social Classes I and II, who went to a public school and who have got a university degree. In contrast, the Welsh CHC members are consistently below the national average on all these counts, in some cases dramatically so. For instance, 28% of the CHC members in Wales are women as against 52% in the North West Thames region; 45% of the Welsh members are professionals or managers as against 69% of the North Thames members; again, while 10% of the former have been to public school and 20% to university, the equivalent figures for the latter arc 38% and 37% respectively. In contrast, Wales is remarkable for having the highest proportion — far higher than the North West Thames region — of members who went to grammar schools: almost two-thirds of the total. In other words, two different kinds of societies have produced two recognisably different sets of representatives, even though the difference is one of degree rather than kind: to exaggerate, the Welsh grammar-school patriarchy sets a different imprint on its CHCs than the cosmopolitan matriarchy of the metropolis.

Again, it is possible to pick out a group of regions (Figure 2.2) — Mersey, the Northern, Trent, Wales and West Midlands — where an above-average proportion of CHC members are blue-collar in line with what might be expected from the social and industrial geography of the country. In contrast, the regions where blue-collar representation is below the national average — the four Thames regions, the South Western and Wessex — fall into two categories, the metropolitan and the rural, both of whose characteristics differ from those in the first, above-average group.

But the relationships involved are complex and the processes by which

Figure 2.2 Regional variations in the proportion of blue collar workers

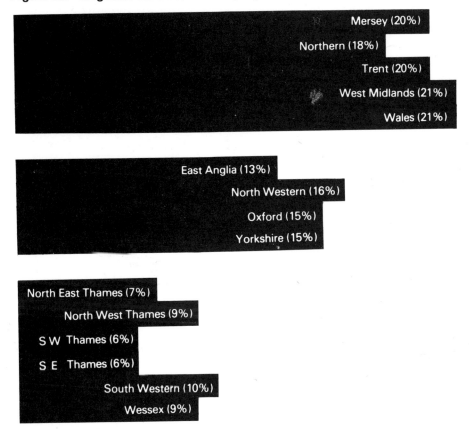

Mersey (20%)

Northern (18%)

Trent (20%)

West Midlands (21%)

Wales (21%)

East Anglia (13%)

North Western (16%)

Oxford (15%)

Yorkshire (15%)

North East Thames (7%)

North West Thames (9%)

S W Thames (6%)

S E Thames (6%)

South Western (10%)

Wessex (9%)

the characteristics of the community leave their imprint on the characteristics of the CHC members are neither direct nor straightforward: certainly our evidence only permits speculation on the nature of the social mechanisms involved. Comparing the rankings of the age structure of the regional populations and of their CHC members (Table 2.8), there is some evidence of correspondence between the two: at the extremes, the Oxford region has the youngest population and the youngest CHC membership while, at the other end of the scale, the South Western region has one of the oldest population and nearly the highest proportion of CHC members over 65. Again, the age structures of Wales and the West Midlands are echoed, if with some slight distortion, in the age profile of their CHC members. However, the relationship is far from consistent: thus while the South West Thames region ranks high for its proportion of the population over 65, its CHC members rank low on this criterion. This lack of any systematic relationship is evident also in the variations in the ratio between men and women in the different regions (Table 1A). In the population as a whole, the range of variations in this ratio is small: the proportion of men ranges from 47% to 49.5%. But among CHC members the regional variations range from 48% to 71%. So the explanation ought, perhaps, to be sought in differences in social structure — meaning by this the local political traditions and social networks which mediate the recruitment of people into the arena of public and voluntary service — rather than the familiar, standard socio-economic variables.

The need for caution in drawing conclusions about the CHC membership from such socio-economic variables can be further illustrated (Tables 3A to 5A). For instance, East Anglia and Oxford have an almost identical social-class profile. But while 61% of the Oxford region's members had some form of further education, only 52% in East Anglia fell into this category (a difference related, perhaps, to the age structure of the two regions: Oxford, as noted above, is an exceptionally young region and, given the expansion of further education in recent decades, it is not surprising to find a relationship between age structure and educational experience). But when it comes to the proportion of CHC members who went to a public school, the position is reversed and the percentage is higher in East Anglia than in Oxford. This is to stress the obvious — but often neglected point — that social classes are not homogeneous in the experience which they bring to service on CHCs. They are useful analytical categories when comparing CHC members to the population at large. They must not be confused with predictors of how people are likely to behave or even of what values they are likely to bring to their role as representatives. As we shall see subsequently in this chapter, they are spectacularly inaccurate as predictors of political loyalties; many CHC members may be in a representative role precisely because they are unrepresentative of their social class.

Since the CHC membership seems to reflect variations in social and political structure, but emphatically does not mirror the population in a literal or precise sense, it comes as no surprise to find that the differences within regions are even more pronounced (and apparently more arbitrary) than those between them. This indeed is to be expected since the NHS regions are administrative artefacts, rather than communities with any sense of identity or social homogeneity. The proportion of men on individual CHCs ranges from 19% on one council to 73% on another in Trent and from 44% to 89% in the North Western region (Figure 2.3).

Figure 2.3 The range of individual councils within
two regions Percentage of men

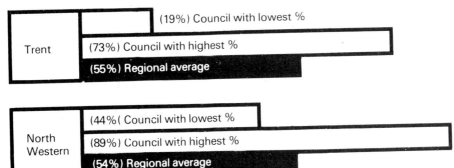

The difference in the regions of the proportion of CHC members who are professionals or managers varies from 44% to 69% ; within Trent, the region with the lowest overall total, the range for individual CHCs is from 27% to 73% ; in the North West Thames, the region with the highest overall total, the range is from 40% to 93% . (Figure 2.4). Moreover, the asymmetry in the social mix of CHC members is exaggerated even further when the analysis switches from the regions to the individual CHCs. In ten out of the 15 regions, there are CHCs with no working class representatives. In contrast, there is no council in our sample without middle-class representation and, perhaps more remarkably still, only one with a majority of working class members[7].

Figure 2.4 The range of individual CHCs within two regions
Percentage of professional and managerial occupations

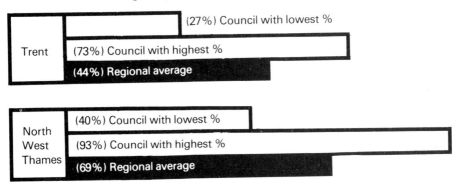

Given these remarkable differences between individual CHCs, it is tempting to concentrate on these in the analysis of the survey results. It is at this level, after all, that the texture of the local community — in all its various strands, from social composition to political structure — might be expected to have the greatest influence in determining the membership of CHCs: an influence which might well be blurred or totally concealed by aggregating the data. But, for reasons already explained, the available national data does not permit such a micro-analysis. In what follows we concentrate on the 32 CHCs where the response rate was over 80%. These are in no way a sample of the whole. So the information derived from them is used illustratively only: our evidence raises some interesting and intriguing points, and should always be read with this caution in mind.

At the extremes, examining individual CHCs does suggest that they reflect the community which they represent — not in a precise statistical sense, but rather in presenting an exaggerated parody of the stereotype evoked by the names of the relevant district. If one were to reel off the names of Westminster, Kensington and Chelsea, Cambridge and Oxford in one group, and those of Merthyr Tydfil, South Sheffield and Halton in another, it would come as no surprise that the former includes the CHCs with the highest concentration of middle-class members and the latter those with the highest concentration of blue-collar workers. In North East Westminster, Kensington and Chelsea, 93% of the members are in the professional and managerial category; in Halton the equivalent figure is only 35% (to take the two CHCs at the opposite ends of this distribution). But the extent to which CHCs may be a distorting mirror — capturing one aspect of a community and grossly over-emphasising it — is illustrated by the example of Cambridge: there the professionals and managers swept the board to the virtual exclusion of white-collar workers. These are represented by only one member although it would be difficult to argue that Cambridge — anymore than Westminster, Kensington and Chelsea — is so disproportionately lacking in such workers. More generally, there seems to be no precise or direct correspondence between the social class composition of the population and that of the CHCs; one reason for this — the political structure of the communities — will emerge in the following section.

Turning to another aspect of the communities being represented, their age structure, the evidence again tends to support the "distorting-mirror" interpretation (Table 2.9). Taking the six CHCs with the highest proportion of members over 65, in five out of six cases the local community also contains an above average number of people above the retirement age. But taking the six CHCs with the lowest proportion of members over 65, the picture is somewhat different. While the relevant communities tend to be at or slightly below the national average for the proportion of over 65s in the population all the CHCs are dramatically below the survey average for members over 65. So CHCs are, at best, flawed and inconsistent reflections of the communities they speak for and, at worst, grotesque parodies of the social composition of the population being represented.

But the evidence so far presented may exaggerate these similarities. For the discussion has hitherto concentrated on reviewing only those aspects of the CHC membership which is relevant to the "mirror of the community" theory of representation. To the extent that this is an inadequate theory — and, as such, a misleading guide to policy — so it is necessary to look at the CHC membership in the light of other concepts of representation. If the CHC membership is examined from a different point of view — in terms of the representation of the community not in an atomistic sense of the individuals who compose it but as a bundle of interests and a complex network of groups — then a different picture may emerge. So it is to this analysis that the next section turns.

Groups, links and networks

In analysing the composition of the CHC membership in terms of the representation of groups within the community, there are a number of difficulties. Like the word "representative", the concept of "representation" is slippery and elusive. Someone who is elected to the CHC by a particular group may well represent that interest in a different way from someone who merely happens to be a member of that group: in the former instance, he or she may well feel themselves to be a spokesman for his or her constituency, while in the latter case the relationship may be much more tenuous, some CHC members may represent groups implicitly, because of shared valued; others may be more explicit in their roles. Examining the representation of groups within the community — by looking, as this section does, at the links between CHC members and voluntary organisations — should not, therefore, be equated with trying to predict the attitudes, far less the behaviour, of the councils.

Like representation, the concept of groups is very much a hold-all. There are, for example, the traditional ways of classifying pressure groups by whether they are self-interested or altruistic, whether they represent the interests of clients and consumers or those of providers and professionals, and so on[8] . A different perspective can be used in categorising groups depending on the view taken of the arena in which they act. For instance, groups can be viewed as actors in a complex political system — the

National Health Service in the context of our discussion — competing for scarce resources, and using the currency of influence and pressure. On this view, the important question is who has or has not got access to the political market. Alternatively the groups can be seen as part of a complex information network. To the extent that representation means seeking, or at least being accessible to, the views of those being represented, so it is important to know where, how and to what extent members of CHCs "plug" into the complex network of organisations within the community. For it is these organisations which are, as it were, the intelligence network of the community — collecting and passing on information, censoring some messages or distorting others. The first is what might be called the competition model; the second might be labelled the co-operative model.

In practice such distinctions — while highly relevant to an analysis of the behaviour of groups — are somewhat less helpful when discussing the extent to which the composition of CHCs reflects the composition of the community. Given that the focus of interest is representation, rather than behaviour [9] , our analysis does not attempt to categorise groups in terms of political and social theory. Instead it looks at the representation of voluntary organisations in the light of the explicit and implicit policy objectives — in so far as these can be discerned — which lay behind the establishment of the CHCs in the first place.

Perhaps the most basic objective of all was, as seen in the previous chapter, to involve as many voluntary organisations as possible: in order to establish more links between the NHS and the community and to encourage interest in, and support for, the service. And, in the event, CHC members turn out to be part of a complex and extended network of such organisations (Table 2.10: this excludes political parties, trade-unions and churches, which are considered separately below). Only 15% of them are not linked to any voluntary organisation, while 20% of them are members of four or more such organisations. The frequency of membership rises with social class: while the excess of middle class members means that the population is not accurately represented in social terms, this does bring with it more contacts with the existing network of organisations.

But the aim in setting up the CHCs was not just to recruit the largest possible number of people with voluntary organisation links. Additionally, the objective was to bias the selection deliberately to ensure representation by proxy for the most vulnerable, and perhaps least articulate, sections of the community. In the outcome, the system of fancy franchises invented to choose voluntary organisation representatives, appears to have worked. The special care groups like the mentally handicapped and the physically disabled are well represented. One-tenth of CHC councillors are members of organisations concerned with mental health, while one-quarter of them are members of organisations concerned with the elderly (Table 2.11). Mere membership does not necessarily imply active involvement and interest. The high proportion of voluntary organisation members on CHCs who hold some position in those organisations is therefore particularly noteworthy, since this implies a more than average degree of commitment. For instance, in the case of members of organisations concerned with the physically disabled, almost two-thirds hold some office.

In trying to involve voluntary organisations in general, as distinct from those specifically concerned with special care groups, the main objective of Ministers and civil servants appears to have been to bring support and knowledge into the NHS: i.e. to encourage more voluntary participation and to plug into the information network of voluntary agencies. Here again, the aim of policy appears to have been successful (Table 2.12): the percentage for the various groups of voluntary organisations are, of course, not mutually exclusive). Almost two-fifth of CHC members are members of — and in turn three quarters of these are office holders in — voluntary organisations which perform some sort of supportive function in the health or personal social service area. Another 17% are associated with the Friends of the Hospital group. Different in their self-interest, but similar in their experience, are the 11% who are members of professional organisations involved in the health or social services and the 13% involved in social work activities like youth clubs, hostels for ex-prisoners and so on.

More heterogeneous still are a further group of voluntary organisations (Table 2.13): those which represent different strands of interests — some very general, others narrowly specific — within the community at large, and not directly or exclusively related to the clientele or problems of the social services. Here, unsurprisingly, the best represented organisations are those with the widest and most general interests: the fact that just over a quarter of the men and women on CHCs are members of such civic organisations — Inner Wheels, Townswomen's Guilds, Round Tables, Rotary Clubs and so on — is of significance, perhaps, only to the extent that it suggests a link with yet another network and another source of information about community views and feelings. Much the same is true of the 24% of CHC members who belong to local community groups like tenants' or ratepayers' associations and amenity groups of all kinds. Membership in all such organisations would suggest active, interested citizens — particularly, as is so often the case, when it is accompanied by office-holding.

Different yet again is another group of organisations: those primarily concerned with immigrants. These could, arguably, have been included in the special care groups category. They have been picked out for separate discussion because they received special mention, as requiring representation, in the DHSS's circular giving instructions to the RHAs. One out of every 20 CHC councillors is a member of such organisations. The significance of this figure is even more difficult to assess than that of the other statistics about membership already quoted. Given the uneven distribution of immigrants throughout the country — which is very much more pronounced than for any of the other sections of the population so far discussed — the total number of CHC councillors associated with the appropriate organisations is less important than their precise location. And it is therefore perhaps most illuminating to look at their distribution in the context of a more general analysis of how the membership of voluntary organisations varies from region to region.

Taking, first, the distribution of members of voluntary organisations concerned with special care groups (Figure 2.5 and Table 6A), it is clear

Figure 2.5 Range of membership of voluntary organisations between regions: special care groups

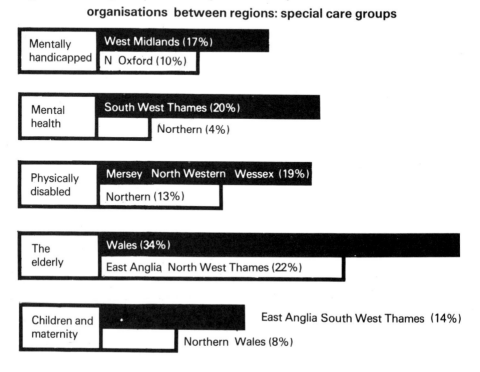

that despite conspicuous variations, there is no region where these particular interests have failed to obtain representation. Assuming that there should be at least one representative for each special care group per CHC, as a very crude criterion of minimum adequacy, this target has been achieved everywhere except for mental health in the Northern region. It must be stressed, however, that even when there are enough members in a region to provide enough representation, there can be no certainty that they will be equally spread between the CHCs within it.

The criterion of one representative for each care group is crude but not arbitrary; it is implicit in the voting arrangements for choosing voluntary organisation members. But if the criterion of minimum adequacy is raised to two representatives for each special care group per CHC, then most regions still satisfy the test for most of the groups: the one apparent exception, the South East Thames, must be ignored for this purpose, since it was the pilot region and the section of the questionnaire asking for details of voluntary organisation membership was not as comprehensive and searching as in the rest of the survey. Even if there had not been a deliberate attempt to guarantee one member for each of these care groups through the system of electing voluntary organisation representatives, it seems as though these groups would still have secured a reasonably widespread presence on CHCs.

Overall, and in line with what might be expected from the national figures, two groups suffer from under-representation in some regions on the criterion of two members per CHC: the mentally ill and mothers and children. For mental health, for example, the differences are large: the South West Thames (20%) has proportionately five times as many CHC members in this category as the Northern (4%) and nearly three times as many as the South Western, North Western regions and Wales. Indeed the Northern region is remarkable for being below the national average for all the special care groups. The reason for this could lie either in the methods of selection adopted or in the ecology of voluntary organisations: it could be that these organisations are thinner on the ground in the Northern than in other regions.

This explanation is consistent with the picture that emerges (Figure 2.6 and Table 7A) from the figures showing the regional distribution of voluntary organisations concerned with health and social services in a general and supportive role. Once again, the Northern region is below the national average for members of organisations like Friends of Hospitals and service or advice giving bodies. In this, the nature of the voluntary organisation system in any given region appears to be more important

41

The politics of consumer representation

Figure 2.6   Range of membership of voluntary organisations between regions: health and social services

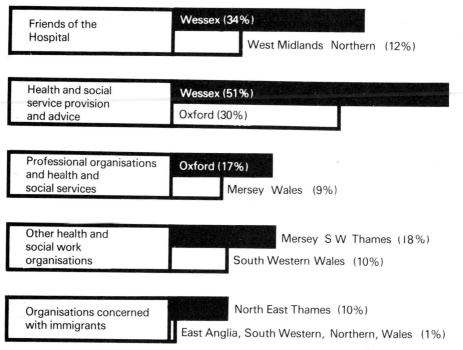

than variations in the methods of choosing CHC members. For example, the South Western region reserved a special constituency for Hospital Friends, but still had a lower proportion (27%) of members in this category than Wessex (34%)[10]. But the question of whether the regional differences in representation accurately mirror the differences in the numbers, degree of commitment and composition of the voluntary organisations in the various regions cannot be answered in the absence of information about the geographical distribution of voluntary activity.

The one instance in which it is possible to see some correspondence, if only in a very rough and ready way, is in the representation of voluntary organisations concerned with immigrants. As pointed out earlier, immigrants are not evenly spread throughout the country, so that considerable regional variations could be predicted. This turns out to be the case. It is no surprise to find that East Anglia, the Northern, South Western and Wales are the parts of the country with the lowest proportion — one per cent — of CHC members associated with immigrant organisations, while at the opposite end of the scale there are North East Thames (10%), West Midlands (9%), South West and North West

Figure 2.7   Range of membership of voluntarv organisations
between regions: civic and community groups

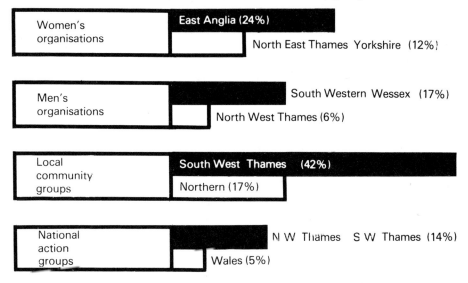

| Women's organisations | East Anglia (24%) | |
| North East Thames Yorkshire (12%) |

| Men's organisations | South Western Wessex (17%) |
| North West Thames (6%) |

| Local community groups | South West Thames   (42%) |
| Northern (17%) |

| National action groups | N W Thames   S W Thames (14%) |
| Wales (5%) |

Thames (both 8%). These groupings, though not necessarily the precise figures, are what might have been anticipated from the distribution of the immigrant population.

Less clear-cut, if rather intriguing, is the regional distribution of CHC members as between what might be called — at the risk of some over-simplification — clubbable and campaigning organisations: between, for example, organisations like Round Tables and those like the Child Poverty Action Group (Figure 2.7 and Table 8A). Intuitively, and speculatively, it seems likely that the former would be stronger in the culture of regions with a strong small town element and the latter would be more visible in the regions of the big conurbations. And, on balance, the trends do appear to be in this direction, though the pattern is less than clear-cut. The three relevant Thames regions have the highest proportion of CHC members belonging to national action groups, while East Anglia, South Western and Trent rank highest for the proportion of members belonging to men's or women's organisations.

So far, in analysing the links between CHC members and the community, the discussion has moved from looking at organisations with a specific health service commitment to those with a vaguer or wider civic interest. But three other categories of organisations have been deliberately excluded: churches, trade-unions and political parties. None of them fit

Figure 2.8   The regional range of church membership and affiliation

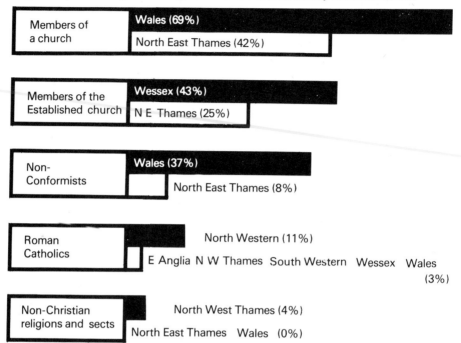

comfortably into the stereotype of voluntary organisations, as conventionally defined within the context of the social services. Their concerns range far beyond the social services and are not necessarily focussed on the needs of the local community. But all are highly relevant when considering the nature of the network of which CHC members are part and the values to which they subscribe. They are also important because of the numbers involved (Table 2.14). Over half the CHC members belong to churches[11]; the same proportion are members of political parties; nearly three in ten are trade-unionists. Moreover, there is a high degree of active commitment as measured by the proportion holding some position or other in the organisations concerned: for instance, over half the members of political parties play some official role.

Once again, there is considerable heterogeneity within the national totals. In the case of religious affiliations this is particularly interesting in that there are variations both as between the proportion of CHC members in different regions who belong to a church and in the denominational composition of the regional totals (Figure 2.8 and Table 9A). Taking the total membership, it is possible to discern yet again the distinction — noted above — between heavily urbanised regions and those with a more mixed pattern of city and country. Church membership is much lower in the former group, the metropolitan regions and the West Midlands, than in the latter, where Wales and Wessex are outstanding for the high proportion of CHC membership with religious affiliations. To judge by this criterion, the CHC membership seems to reflect the regional stereotypes in social traditions — insofar as these overlap with the NHS regions.

This conclusion is further reinforced when the denominational composition of the membership is analysed by region. Not unexpectedly, it is East Anglia, Wessex and the South Western which have the highest proportions of people belonging to the Established Church. Equally unsurprisingly, Wales has more than twice as many non-conformists, proportionately, than any other regions. The above-average representation in Mersey of Roman Catholics — whose membership is, perhaps, of particular interest, given their Church's attitude towards such health service issues as abortion — is predictable: but since the national average is only five per cent, even this does not mean a very strong presence.

Membership of churches is notoriously difficult to define with any precision. But the membership of political parties is a much more precise concept, since it involves paying dues, even though the degree of commitment implied will naturally vary. A CHC councillor is six times more likely to belong to a political party than the average member of the public: the Maud survey, for example, showed that only eight per cent of the electorate claimed to be party members[12]. In other words, and following inevitably from the fact that half of them are nominated by local authorities, the CHC members are drawn disproportionately from the politically active sections of the population.

The CHC members are also untypical in a number of other ways. Compared to the voting patterns in the 1974 General Elections[13], the Labour Party is very much over-represented (Table 2.15). Considering the total CHC membership, almost one-third belong to the Labour Party, one-sixth belong to the Conservative Party and just under one-twentieth belong to the Liberal Party. Considering only those CHC members linked to any political party, well over half are Labour subscribers. This imbalance is, of course, explained by the fact that at the time CHC members were chosen — in 1974, for the most part — the Labour Party controlled far more local authorities than the Conservatives[14]. To anticipate the subsequent discussion of differences between CHC members related to their method of recruitment, party membership is strongly associated with local authority nomination. While four out of five local authority nominees are members of one of the three main parties, almost the same proportion of voluntary organisation nominees are not (Table 2.16). Similarly, while about half the local authority nominees are members of the Labour Party, and a quarter of them are members of the Conservative Party, only one tenth of voluntary organisation nominees belong to each of them. The RHA's nominees tend, like the voluntary organisation nominees, to be apolitical but lean slightly more to the Left.

Analysing party membership another way, by social class (Table 2.17), shows some further differences, and not always in the most predictable direction. Most conspicuously, blue-collar workers are twice as likely to be members of a political party than professionals, managers or white-collar workers: only 24% of the former are not party members, as against 56% and 46% respectively for the other two groups. And, in turn, these blue-collar workers are overwhelmingly Labour supporters. This underlines the crucial importance of the Labour Party in recruiting blue-collar workers into representative positions. But although an overwhelming proportion of blue-collar workers are Labour supporters, they account for only a third of all party members because of their small absolute numbers. The remaining two-thirds are middle class. CHC members from professional and managerial background are just as likely to be Labour as Tory and white-collar workers split in favour of Labour by 56% to 36%.

There are, naturally and unsurprisingly, large variations in party membership as between different regions. Some of these are entirely predictable, and consistent with the balance of social classes (Figure 2.9 and Tables 3A and 10A). the South West Thames, Wessex and South Western are all above the national average in the proportion of middle class men and women and below national average in the percentage of blue-collar workers. They are also, as a neat mirror-image, above average in the proportion of Conservative Party members and below average in the percentage of Labour Party members. So here the stereotype of a middle-class, Church of England and Tory-voting population would seem to hold. Similarly Wales and Trent show precisely the reverse characteristics: comparatively low on middle-class members and comparatively high on working class members, with Tory support below the national average (dramatically so in the case of Wales) and Labour support well above the national average. This neat symmetry does not hold for all regions. For example, the social class profile of Mersey and the Northern regions are virtually identical. But the political profile is very

Figure 2.9 Comparisons of Labour Party membership and social class

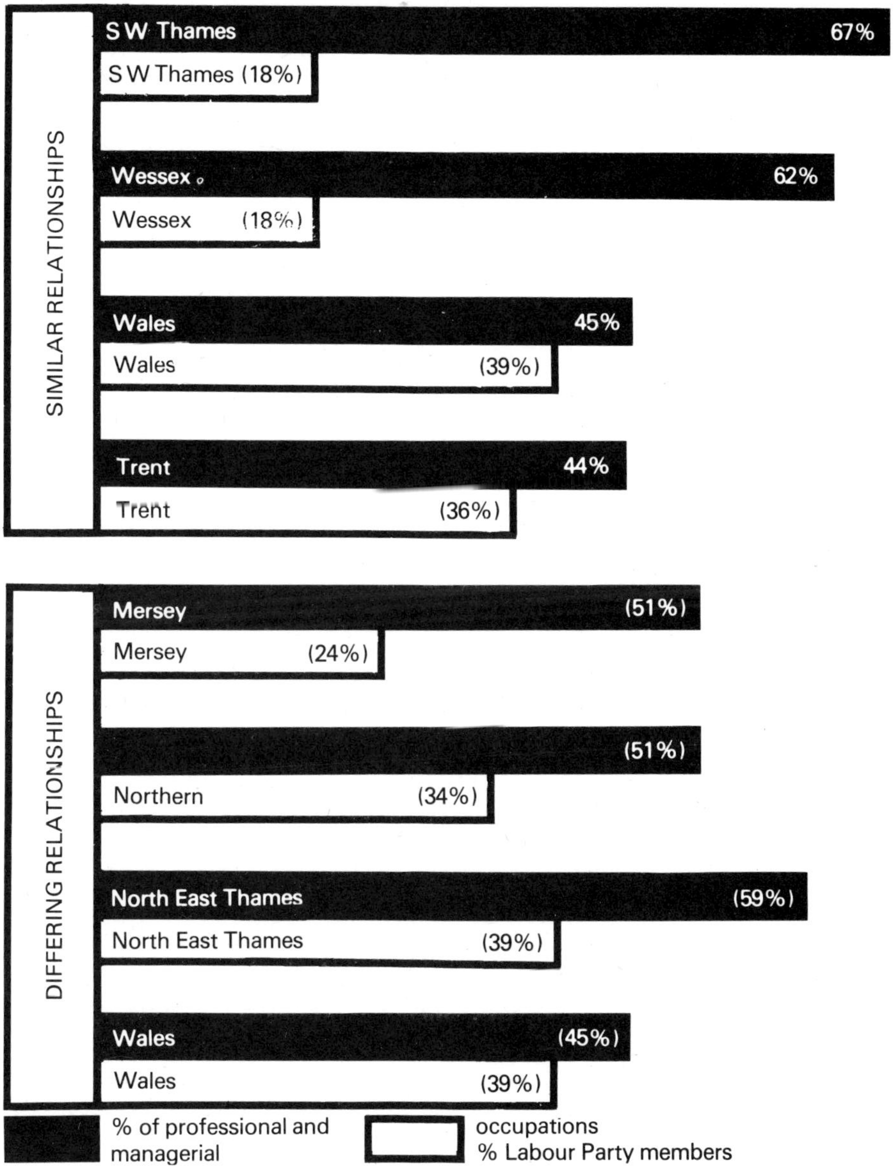

SIMILAR RELATIONSHIPS

S W Thames	67%
S W Thames (18%)	
Wessex	62%
Wessex (18%)	
Wales	45%
Wales (39%)	
Trent	44%
Trent (36%)	

DIFFERING RELATIONSHIPS

Mersey	(51%)
Mersey (24%)	
	(51%)
Northern (34%)	
North East Thames	(59%)
North East Thames (39%)	
Wales	(45%)
Wales (39%)	

■ % of professional and managerial
□ occupations
% Labour Party members

different. In contrast, North East Thames and Wales have identical proportions of Labour Party members, although they differ significantly in social compositions.

The explanation for these puzzling discrepancies, as for some of the anomalies noted in the previous section, could well lie in the social structure of the political systems in the various regions. It is these which, particularly in the case of local authority nominees, are mostly the bodies which select or sieve out those who are to represent the population at large. The lack of correspondence between the community's social characteristics and those of its representatives could therefore be explained both by self-selection among those who participate in public activities and by the nature of the voluntary organisations to which they belong. In the case of the Conservative Party membership, there is a high degree of consistency between social class and political views; there are very few working-class Conservative CHC councillors. In the case of the Labour Party membership, as already noted, there is no such precise correspondence between social class and political affiliations: the scale of blue-collar representation appears to depend as much on the extent to which the relevant local Labour Parties are run by middle-class activists as on the composition of the population at large. If the social structure of the CHCs is biased towards the middle-class, it is partly because it is reflecting a similar bias in the social structure of local Labour parties.

The pattern of party membership in individual CHCs seems to be consistent with this explanation, although it does not justify any very firm conclusions. Taking the CHCs with 40% or more of Conservative Party members — and a response rate above 80% — there are no surprises. They are Blackpool, South Westminster, Kensington and Chelsea, High Wycombe and Canterbury. These are all CHCs with a high proportion of professional and white collar members, and social background is consistent with political loyalty. In contrast, when considering the CHCs where Labour Party members predominate, it at once becomes apparent that the social composition of the community is not only a poor predictor of political loyalty but is frequently inconsistent with it. The CHCs with 40% or more of Labour Party members range from Merthyr Tydfil, which has twice the national average of blue-collar workers, to North Camden, with a third of the national average.

Overall, members of the Labour Party are — as might be expected from the national figures — in a much stronger position to influence the policies of individual CHCs than are members of the Conservative Party. Taking the 155 CHCs with a response rate of above 60%, in only two of them are Conservative Party members in a majority while, as noted above, there are 21 CHCs where Labour Party members are in this position. The contrast is further confirmed by those CHCs where members of one political party are in a dominating position, even though they do not command a majority. In only nine CHCs do the Conservatives have between 40% and 50% of the total membership, while the equivalent figure for Labour is 19. Again, at the opposite end of the scale, there are only two CHCs where Labour is unrepresented, while there are 12 where the Conservatives are unrepresented (heavily concentrated in Wales). These figures, like those discussed earlier, should not of course be equated with assertions about the political dispositions of the CHCs councils as a whole: it could well be that those councillors who are not members of any political party would show a different pattern in their political orientations than the activists. But they do show the extent to which the CHC network is intertwined with — and part of — the already existing political network.

Once again the CHCs appear as something of a distorting mirror: exaggerating the political domination of whatever party happens to be in control of the most local authorities, just as they exaggerate the social composition of the population being represented. Their political complexion may alter with changes in local government politics; the selection procedure's built-in bias towards exaggerating political swings is, however, likely to persist.

Representative competence and public persons

Most discussions of the role of the consumer in health care systems tend to adopt, if only implicitly, one of two models. On the one hand, there is the model of the consumer as the omniscient shopper, able to distinguish between good and bad products [15]. On the other hand, there is the model of the consumer as an idiot child in need of protection against his own ignorance [16]. The first tends to lead to an advocacy of a free market approach to the provision of health care; the second is associated with the advocacy of comprehensive planning. In turn, each of these views has implications for any analysis of consumer representatives in terms of their competence for the role.

For competence can, in this context, have two different meanings related to the view taken of the consumer's position in the health care system. If the consumer is thought of as a shopper able to make his own decisions, then the representative's skill lies in his abilities as a spokesman: he will act just as the consumer would have done, if only the latter had the time or the required experience in using the machinery of representation. If the consumer is thought of as an idiot child, then the representative's skill will lie in possessing knowledge (or the trained capacity to acquire knowledge): his role will be that of a guardian who has to discern, define and voice those interests which the consumer may not be aware of.

Like all models, these present an over-simplified picture of reality. In practice, the situation of the consumer — and of his representative — is more complex. But for the purposes of analysis, it is helpful to distinguish between competence as experience in representation and competence as experience in fields of expertise relevant to the special interests of the health service. This section, therefore, examines CHC members in terms of their experience of, first, representative roles and, second, of the health service.

The most obvious measure of experience in representation is membership of local authorities. This is also an indication of the extent to which the CHC are linked to the local authority system and thus satisfy one of the original aims of policy in setting them up: to encourage greater co-operation between health and local authority services. This was, as noted earlier, one of the reasons why half the CHC members were put into the gift of the relevent local authorities: and this method of nomination explains, in turn, why almost two-fifths of CHC members are also local authority councillors. Overwhelmingly (Table 2.18) local authorities have put their own members on to the CHCs. Over four-fifths of their nominees are local authority councillors. In contrast, only six per cent of voluntary organisation nominees and eight per cent of the regional health authority nominees are local councillors, and even these modest totals slump heavily — to two and three per cent respectively — if parish councillors are excluded. Further, the local authority nominees have also had far more past experience as councillors than those drawn from the other two sources. If past membership is taken into account, then the proportion of local authority nominees with experience of local government rises to 89% (Table 2.19). As so often, there are considerable regional variations. In some regions local authorities appear to nominate their own members almost without exception: Oxford, East Anglia, Wales and Wessex. In others, the North West Thames and the West Midlands, local authorities have given respectively two fifths and a quarter of their seats to non-councillors. In addition, local authorities in some regions — notably the North Western — have rewarded past councillors with membership of

CHCs. There are regional differnces, as well, in the kind of local authorities represented by the councillors (Figure 2.10 and Table 11A). This largely reflects the structure of local government, although it may also be influenced by the apportionment of CHC seats as between the different levels. For instance, there is a higher proportion of parish councillors in the more rural regions like East Anglia and the South Western than elsewhere. Inevitably, too, there are fewer county councillors in the metropolitan regions than in the rest of the country: interestingly, the Greater London Council is barely represented.

Figure 2.10   Range of regional distribution of local authority councillors

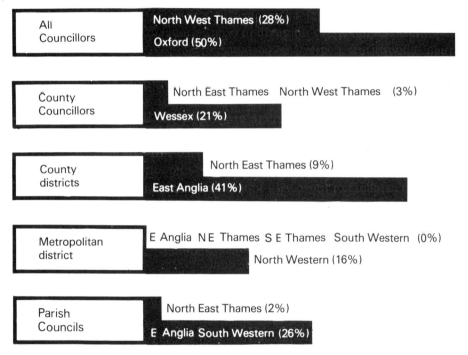

Experience in the performance of public roles — and thus, by implication, some competence as representational spokesmen — cannot be measured by service on local authorities alone (and indeed it may legitimately be objected that experience does not necessarily guarantee competence, anyway). There are a great many other public roles which might be expected to create the self-confidence or provide the training required for representation. To what extent, then, are CHC members drawn from the existing reservoir of "public persons" — i.e. those who are already within the established network — and to what degree have they been fished from a new pool?

In fact (Table 2.20), well over a third of CHC members are emphatically "private" persons in that they are not members of any public bodies on our check list (magistrates, school governors, co-opted members of local authority committees, members of tribunals or members of consultative councils of nationalised industries). A further two-fifths hold only one such position. At the other end of the scale, there are six per cent who hold three or more of these positions, and thus conform to the stereotype of the universal committee man or woman.

The multiple office holders are, perhaps predictably, heavily concentrated among the local authority nominees. Four times as many voluntary organisation nominees as local authority nominees have no position at all. Again, only four per cent of the former hold three or more positions as against nine per cent of the latter. Regional Health Authority nominees are different yet again: they resemble the voluntary organisation members in that they include a high proportion who hold no position at all, but have as high a percentage of those holding three or more offices as the local authority category.

Perhaps the most important single reason why local authority members are so different is that they tend, overwhelmingly, to be school governors (Tables 2.21 and 12A). This turned out to be by far the most important item in our catalogue of public positions: over half the total number of offices held by CHC members fell into this category. In particular, four-fifths of local authority nominees are also school governors, as against a quarter and two-fifths respectively for the other two sets of CHC members. One sixth of local authority and RHA nominees were also magistrates, but the proportion of voluntary organisation nominees was one in fourteen. Overall, then, the public persons on CHCs tend to be recruited from, and be mainly experienced in, local government.

But representational competence cannot, of course, be assessed exclusively by the number of public offices held. Also relevant is the background and experience of CHC members in activities with a direct bearing on health care. Some of these have already been discussed in the context of voluntary organisation membership: participation in voluntary organisations directly involved in the NHS will obviously provide relevant experience. Equally, the professional qualifications and occupation of CHC members have a bearing on their representational capacity, and we subsequently present data on this point. First, however, we look at the record of CHC councillors in a hybrid capacity: as members of health authorities where they might be expected to gain both representational competence and knowledge about the specific concerns of the health care system.

In all, some two-fifths of CHC members have had previous experience on health authorities (Table 2.22). And within this national total, there are regional variations both in the proportion of CHC members with experience of any kind and in the sources of that experience. The range in the proportion of CHC members who have served on any kind of health authority is from just under a third in the West Midlands to half in Wessex. And within these regional totals there are considerable differences in the types of health authorities on which CHC members have served. Overall, the largest single category is service on local authority health committees: here the range is from 15% of all CHC members in the West Midlands to 29% in the North Western regions. Next come those who had been on a Hospital Management Committee in the NHS previous to reorganisation: about a fifth of all CHC members in the North, Wessex and the South Western, as against around a tenth in Mersey, Oxford and the metropolitan regions. It is the combination of a high proportion of CHC members with service both on HMCs and on Hospital House Committees (while these existed) which swells the total experience in both Wessex, the South Western, and to a lesser degree, the Northern regions. These regions are distinctive for the high concentration of NHS experience among their CHC members. This is not to argue that the CHCs will necessarily be more competent in their role as a result: it has been claimed that experience on an HMC, while providing relevant background knowledge, could persuade CHC members to be excessively management-minded [17]. In any event, CHCs run no risk of domination by former members of regional or teaching hospital boards: in all, only four per cent of members have been on either.

There are conspicuous variations between CHC members nominated by different methods (Table 2.23). Over three quarters of the voluntary organisation nominees have never served on a health committee of any kind, as against 50% of local authority and 45% of RHA nominees. But the experience of the local authority members was heavily concentrated on LA health committees, while that of the RHA members was on HMCs. The one-sixth of RHA nominees accounted for a disproportionate share of experience in running hospital and general practitioner services in the old NHS.

The picture changes yet again when the occupational background of CHC members is examined. In total, 13% of CHC members have occupations directly relevant to the NHS: that is, they are either doctors, nurses or ancillary health service staff (Table 2.24). There are a further 11% with relevant experience in the social services: social workers, full-time workers in voluntary organisations and similar jobs. Finally, there is a category of those with jobs which give them an experience either of public services or of social problems, and often of both: teachers, clergy, central or local government staff. Two-fifths of all CHC members are drawn from what might be called the social services and other public services sector. In addition, there are some CHC members who have the appropriate qualifications for this category, but do not appear to have used them at work (Table 13A). When the two-fifths of CHC members who fall into this broad social and public service category are analysed by their sponsoring bodies, it becomes clear that those nominated by voluntary organisations make up in occupational experience for what they lack in representational experience of service on public bodies (Table 2.25). While 56% of all voluntary organisation nominees have a relevant occupational background, the equivalent figures for the local authority and RHA nominees are respectively 29% and 45%.

So far the analysis has treated all CHC members as though they were totally undifferentiated in their roles. In one important respect, this is wrong. The responsibilities of a CHC chairman are wider than those of other members, and he or she is more likely to shape the style of any individual CHC. And, as it turns out, the profile of CHC chairmen is different from that of the rest of the Membership (Table 2.26). Most conspicuously, the slight preponderance of men in the total membership turns into male dominance when it comes to the chairmanships: almost four-fifths are men. Again, voluntary organisation nominees get less than their share of chairmanships than either of the other two categories: 18% of the chairmen are sponsored by voluntary organisations as against 29% who come from the one-sixth of members nominated by RHAs. Chairmen are also more likely to be public persons — magistrates, school governors and so on — than the average CHC member. Lastly, to conclude the catalogue of differences, almost one-third of chairmen have a university degree as against only a fifth of all CHC members, and there is a slight over-representation of the middle classes and a slight under-representation of blue-collar workers among the chairmen. In short, there is a tendency for the differences between the CHC membership and the population at large to become more pronounced and exaggerated when the chairmen are compared with the rank and file of members.

Do methods of selection matter?

The most obvious way in which CHCs differ from other experiments in consumer representation — in the nationalised industries, for example — is in the methods adopted for selecting their members. In particular, the decision to permit voluntary organisations to elect their own representatives — which, as seen in the previous chapter, was an almost accidental invention under pressure from Parliament and other bodies — meant a sharp break with past practices. Even though everyone stressed that the nominees of voluntary organisations were not to be regarded as representatives in a strict sense — they were, it was emphasised, to see themselves as having a collective responsibility for all consumers and not just for a particular group — this method did mark them out as different from the members of, say, a consultative committee attached to a nationalised industry who had been picked by civil servants and lacked any sort of constituency in the community. Was all this trouble worthwhile? Is the whole cumbersome system of selection justified by the results it has achieved or should it be scrapped in favour of a return to the traditional methods of nomination by civil servants or health authorities? These questions are not only important for the future of the CHCs themselves. They are also relevant for future policy-making about consumer representation in general, to the extent that the experience of the CHCs may be taken either as a model or as a warning.

In one sense, these questions do not permit any answer. If they are taken to mean "which methods of selection produces the most effective CHC members", then it would be futile to pretend that answers can be found in their social, educational or political backgrounds. But if the question is whether the different methods of selection produce different types of men and women — and therefore introduce elements of variety and experience which would otherwise be lacking — then it is possible, on the basis of the data collected in our survey, to come to some conclusions about the methods of appointment.

Some of the differences between CHC members, related to the way in which they were chosen, have already been touched on. But it is worth recalling and underlining what is the most significant of these: the CHC members nominated by voluntary organisations are different from the rest — and in particular from local authority nominees — in that they come from a pool of people which might otherwise not be tapped. A new method of selection does appear to have drawn members from a new source. The qualities which these CHC members bring to their role is not so much experience in public representation (the strength of the local authority members) or experience in health service management (the contribution of RHA nominees) but experience of work relevant to the substantive interests of the health and other social services.

But extending the range of recruitment was only one of the objectives of policy in involving the voluntary organisations. A more important consideration was to ensure representation for certain, specific and particularly vulnerable care groups, and — as already seen — this aim has indeed been achieved. But our earlier analysis did not distinguish, in discussing the representation of the various special care groups, the composition of the representatives by their nominating bodies. Would these care groups still be represented on CHCs even if the voluntary organisation nominees did not exist? The answer is that if all these members were suddenly to disappear through a trap-door, there would still be representation for the vulnerable — but it would be less strong (Table 2.27). The representation of the mentally handicapped and ill, the physically disabled and mothers and children would be more than halved. Only in the case of the elderly, where a high proportion of local authority councillors have links with the appropriate voluntary organisations, would there still be a strong membership. More generally, the links with the voluntary organisation network would be weakened but would not disappear. Unsurprisingly, both local authority and RHA nominees belong to fewer voluntary organisations than the members sponsored by the voluntary organisations themselves, but even so their links are far from negligible: 30% of local authority and 33% of RHA nominees belong to three or more voluntary organisations, as against 46% of voluntary organisation nominees (Table 2.28).

Turning from the voluntary organisation nominees to those of the RHA, it is again possible to test whether the aims of policy were achieved. For the policy objectives were, to some extent, explicitly laid down. One aim was to ensure the presence of members "with a special knowledge of health services", acquired by service on NHS management bodies[18]. This has been achieved. Not only are the RHA nominees more qualified in these terms than other CHC members, but the fund of previous experience in NHS management would be much reduced in their absence. Another objective was to guarantee the presence of "bodies such as women's organisations, trade unions, the Churches and youth and immigrant bodies, who might not otherwise be appointed". In this respect, reserving one-sixth of the places for RHA nominees was superfluous. All the organisations named would have been well represented (Table 2.29) if there had not been a single RHA nominee. For example, a strong trade-union presence is assured by the local authority nominees. And even in the case of immigrant organisations, RHA nominees represent only one-seventh of the total number of representatives. It may be that in specific CHCs the RHA nominees fill what would otherwise be gaps in the pattern of representation for these groups; however, the national figures suggest that they are at most icing on the cake of representation.

As far as the local authority nominees are concerned, it is clear that their presence on CHCs is important for one particular reason (ignoring the general argument for encouraging co-operation by cross-member-ships). This is that, but for them, there would be hardly any representation of blue-collar workers on CHCs (Table 2.30), and that white-collar workers would also be somewhat under-represented. Even among local authority nominees, CHC members from a blue-collar background are in a minority — less than a quarter of them can be so classified — and are outnumbered by the middle-class members. But the excess of such middle-class members is less pronounced than for voluntary organisation and RHA nominees: these last are easily the most "top-heavy" in terms of their social class composition. Of local authority nominees more are men, more are over 65, and fewer have been to university or have any qualifications. If CHCs were entirely nominated by local authorities and RHAs, they would be even more male-dominated than they are already: it is the fact that a majority of voluntary organisation nominees are women which helps to prevent the balance of the sexes from being more skewed that it is at present.

To sum up, it would therefore appear that, to the limited extent that it is possible to apply any sort of criteria to the aims of policy, they have been successful. A variety of methods has managed to create a greater diversity among the members — with a wider representation of social experience, occupational background, interest groups and public service know-how — than might otherwise have been the case.

1 Notably, W.L. Guttsman *The British Political Elite* Macgibbon & Kee 1968. But see also Richard Rose *The Problem of Party Government* Macmillan 1974 and Philip Stanworth and Anthony Giddens (eds.) *Elites and power in British Society* Cambridge University Press 1974.

2 In all analyses of the range of variation between CHCs, only those with a response rate of more than 60% are included. But when the focus narrows on the particular characteristics of individual CHCs, we have for the most part concentrated on those with a response of more than 80%.

3 On sending out our questionnaire, we got a number of indignant protests from women members of CHCs who objected to having their social class determined by the occupation of the head of household. This was done, of course, in order to make our information comparable with that in the Census.

4 Committee on the Management of Local Government *Vol.2 The Local Government Councillor* HMSO 1967.

5 Information about the membership of NHS authorities before reorganisation is remarkably scarce: the only source is Mary Stewart *Unpaid public service* Fabian Occasional Paper No.3 1964; post-1973, the situation is little better, but see Rudolf Klein 'NHS committees' *New Society* 6 September 1973.

6 K. Prewitt, *The Recruitment of political leaders: a study of citizen politicians* Bobbs-Merrill 1970. This American study found that "socio-economic differences between councilmen parallel the differences between the communities in which they are elected" p.36.

7 All these statements are based (see note 2 above) on CHCs with a response of 60% or above. This means that there may well in practice be more than one CHC with a working class majority. To repeat our earlier warning, this analysis should be read as an indication of the bias of the system of selection, not as a precise description of the outcome.

8 For a review of the pressure group literature, see Graeme C. Moodie and Gerald Studdert-Kennedy *Opinions, Publics and Pressure Groups* Allen & Unwin 1970.

9 For a behavioural approach to the analysis of representation and a critique of the assumption that activity can be deduced from composition, see Heinz Eulau and Kenneth Prewitt *Labyrinths of Democracy* Bobbs-Merrill 1973.

10 The setting-up process is described in Rudolf Klein and Janet Lewis 'Community Health Councils: The Early Days' *Health and Social Service Journal* 7 December 1974.

11 The problems of giving precise meaning to Church "membership" are well-known and, since we are not particularly concerned about intensity of commitment or frequency of attendance, we did not try to restrict the self-definition of respondents.

12 Committee on the Management of Local Government *Vol.3 The Local Government Elector* HMSO 1967 Table 202. A more recent survey has suggested that only five per cent of the electorate are individual party members: see Richard Rose *Politics in England Today* Faber & Faber 1974. Indeed the assymetry between the representation of Labour and Conservative party members among CHC councillors becomes more remarkable still when account is taken of the disparity in numbers between them: see, David Butler and Michael Pinto-Duschinsky *The British General Election of 1970* Macmillan 1970, where it is estimated that there were then about 350,000 Labour and 1,600,000 Conservative individual party members.

13 This is true whether the February or the October 1974 General Election figures are considered. This comparison seems more sensible than relating the political affiliations of the CHC members to the voting preferences shown

in public opinion polls at the time of their nomination: an exercise in spurious pedantry.

14 Section 6 (2) of the National Health Service (Community Health Councils) Regulations 1973 — S.I. 1973 No.2217 — provides that those local authority nominees who are also elected councillors shall cease to be CHC members if they lose their seat. The results of the May 1976 local elections, which saw a large swing to the Conservatives, could therefore be reflected in a changed CHC membership with different political affiliations. In practice some local authorities have re-nominated deposed members.

15 Milton Friedman *Capitalism and Freedom* University of Chicago Press 1962 Chapter IX.

16 Brian Abel-Smith *Value for money in health services* Heinemann 1976. See especially p.41. In taking Friedman and Abel-Smith as the exponents of the stereotype extremes, we have over-simplified but not, we believe, distorted their views.

17 The tendency of lay members of health authorities to take up an excessively "managerial" stance has been criticised in a series of reports, starting with the Ely inquiry: Rudolf Klein 'Accountability in the National Health Service' *Political Quarterly* October/December 1971. For a more recent illustration of this point, see *Report of Committee of Enquiry, St. Augustine's Hospital, Chartham, Canterbury* South East Thames Regional Health Authority 1976. But much of the criticism begs the question of whether it is the role itself or the experience which is decisive in shaping attitudes: in other words, we don't really know whether this is a problem of structure or function. The reorganisation of the NHS was based on the assumption that it was a problem of structure; it is perhaps somewhat less easy to be confident about this in the light of subsequent experience.

18 NHS Reorganisation Circular HRC(74)4 Para.17.

2.1   AGE DISTRIBUTIONS COMPARED

	Total CHC Survey %	'Maud' Local authority councillors[1] %	Total population of England & Wales (excluding under 15 year olds)[2] %
Under 25	1	4	19
25–34	9		16
35–44	18	15	15
45–54	29	26	16
55–64	28	31	16
65 and over	14	23	18
Not stated	1	1	—
	100% (N = 3,796)	100% (N = 3,970)	100%

Source:
1. Committee on the Management of Local Government vol. 2 'The local government councillor'. HMSO 1967 p. 16.
2. Census 1971. Age, marital condition and general tables. Table 9 England and Wales. HMSO 1975.

2.2   SEX DISTRIBUTIONS COMPARED

	Total CHC Survey %	'Maud' Local authority councillors[1] %	Hospital management committee members[2] %	Total population of England and Wales[3] %
Males	57	88	72	49
Females	43	12	28	51
	100% (N = 3,796)	100% (N = 3,970)	100% (N = 117)	

1. Committee on the Management of Local Government vol. 2 'The local government councillor'. HMSO 1967 p. 50.
2. Royal Commission on Local Government in England 1960–1969. Volume III p. 135. HMSO 1969.
3. Census 1971. Age, marital condition and general tables. Table 9 England and Wales. HMSO 1975.

2.3   SOCIAL CLASS DISTRIBUTIONS COMPARED

	Total CHC Survey Males	Total CHC Survey Females	Total CHC Survey	'Maud' Local authority councillors[1]	Total population of England & Wales
	%	%	%	%	%
Professional	18	18	18	9	4.9
Intermediate	32	43	36	48	18
Non-manual	29	25	27	13	10.2
Skilled manual	17	7	13	17	35.7
Semi-skilled manual	1	0	1	7	16.1
Unskilled manual	1	1	1	3	6.5
Unclassified	3	7	5	3	8.3
	100% (N = 2,150)	100% (N = 1,634)	100% (N = 3,796)	100% (N = 3,970)	100%

(The social class classification was based on the occupation of the head of the household.)

1. Committee on the Management of Local Government, vol. 2. 'The local government councillor'. HMSO 1967 p. 35.
2. Census 1971 (10% sample). Household composition tables, Part III, Table 46. England and Wales. HMSO 1975.

2.4   MARITAL STATUS

Married	Single	Widowed Divorced Separated	Not stated	
3,155	322	298	21	(N = 3,796)
83%	8%	8%	1%	100%

NUMBER OF CHILDREN UNDER 16

No children under 16	One child	Two children	Three children	Four children	Five children or more	Not stated	
2,471	471	443	216	63	19	113	(N = 3,796)
65%	12%	12%	6%	2%	1%	3%	100%

PLACE OF RESIDENCE

Resident in the district	Not resident in the district	Not stated	
3,423	369	4	(N = 3,796)
90%	10%		100%

LENGTH OF RESIDENCE IN THE DISTRICT

Under 5 years	5—9 years	10—14 years	15 years and over	Not stated	
328	394	363	2,296	42	(N = 3,423)
10%	12%	11%	67%	1%	100%

2.5   SCHOOLS ATTENDED SINCE THE AGE OF 11

	%
Elementary	30
Comprehensive	1
Secondary modern	10
Grammar/Technical	51
Public school/private school	26
Others	5
Not stated	1
	124% (N = 3,796)

2.6   FULL-TIME FURTHER EDUCATION

	%
No full-time further education	47
University	23
Polytechnic/CAT	4
Teacher training college/college of education	7
Technical college/college of further education	11
Other further education	5
Not stated	9
	106% (N = 3,796)

2.7 EMPLOYMENT STATUS

	Total CHC survey	'Maud' local authority councillors[1]	Total population[2]	Males in survey	Males in population	Females in survey	Females in population
	%	%	%	%	%	%	%
Working full-time	51	66	49	73	74	23	26
Working part-time	11	5	9	4	3	19	15
Working in unpaid capacity	10	not available	not available	3	not available	20	not available
Retired	17	20	13	21	12	11	14
Full-time housewife	16	7	29	0	11	36	46
Not in employment	4	1		2		6	
Not stated	1	1	—	1	—	1	
	110% (N = 3,796)	100% (N = 3,970)	100%	104% (N = 2,150)	100%	116% (N = 1,634)	100%

1. Committee on the Management of Local Government Vol. 2 p. 19. HMSO 1967.
2. Social Trends. No. 6. HMSO 1975. Table 3.2 for GB and UK not England and Wales.

2.8 **POPULATION DISTRIBUTIONS RANKED: THE CHCs COMPARED WITH THE TOTAL POPULATION IN EACH REGION**

	15—44		45—64		65+	
	CHC survey	Total popula- tion	CHC survey	Total popula- tion	CHC survey	Total popula- tion
East Anglia	8	5	13	12	1	5
Mersey	12	4	5	2	4	10
Northern	11	5	8	2	2	10
North East Thames	4	5	11	2	8	8
North West Thames	2	2	14	12	9	13
North Western	6	10	5	2	9	5
Oxford	1	1	14	15	15	15
South East Thames	10	14	2	2	12	1
South West Thames	3	12	11	2	12	3
South Western	14	15	3	2	2	1
Trent	8	5	3	2	9	10
Wales	15	12	1	1	4	5
Wessex	12	10	5	12	6	3
West Midlands	5	2	9	2	12	13
Yorkshire	6	5	10	2	6	8

Ranking: 1 = region with the highest proportion in the relevant category. See Table 2A for basic data.

2.9 COMPARISONS BETWEEN THE PROPORTION OF OVER 65s
ON CHCs AND THE TOTAL POPULATION OF THEIR DISTRICT[1]

The 6 CHCs with the highest % of over 65's

	% of 65+ in the CHC membership	% of 65+ in the population of the district
East Dorset	33	27
Cornwall	30	23
North Staffordshire	26	16
Weston-super-Mare	24	26
North Devon	21	25
South Sheffield	21	19

The 6 CHCs with the lowest % of over 65s

North East Westminster, Kensington and Chelsea	0	17
Harrow	3	18
Bury	4	17
Halton	4	14
Hounslow	5	18
North Nottingham	5	17
National figures	14	18

1. CHCs with a response rate of 80% or more.

2.10 **THE DISTRIBUTION OF THE MEMBERSHIP OF VOLUNTARY ORGANISATIONS BY SOCIAL CLASS**

	The number of organisations						
	None	One	Two	Three	Four	Five or more	
	%	%	%	%	%	%	
Professional and managerial	10	24	24	18	11	12	100% (N = 2,054)
White collar	17	26	24	15	9	8	100% (N = 1,029)
Blue collar	29	28	19	12	6	7	100% (N = 542)
Not classified	—	—	—	—	—	—	(N = 171)
All social classes	15	25	23	16	10	10	100% (N = 3,796)

2.11 **MEMBERSHIP OF VOLUNTARY ORGANISATIONS INVOLVED WITH SPECIAL CARE GROUPS**

Organisations concerned primarily with: —	Individuals belonging to these organisations (N = 3,796)		Individuals holding a position in these organisations (N = total membership in relevant organisation)	
The mentally handicapped	490	13%	286	58%
Mental health	373	10%	176	47%
The physically disabled	600	16%	392	65%
The elderly	942	25%	599	64%
Children and maternity	371	10%	222	60%

2.12 MEMBERSHIP OF VOLUNTARY ORGANISATIONS CONCERNED WITH HEALTH OR SOCIAL SERVICES

	Individuals belonging to these organisations (N = 3,796)		Individuals holding a position in these organisations (N = total membership in relevant organisation)	
Friends of the Hospital	639	17%	297	46%
Organisations providing health or social services or advice (e.g. Red Cross, St. Johns, WRVS, FPA, Councils of Social Service, Marriage Guidance)	1,485	39%	1,123	76%
Professional organisations involved in health or social services	428	11%	142	33%
Any other health or social work organisation	511	13%	175	34%

2.13   MEMBERSHIP OF CIVIC, COMMUNITY
OR ACTION GROUPS

	Individuals belonging to these organisations (N = 3,796)		Individuals holding a position in these organisations (N = total membership in relevant organisation)	
Women's organisations	645	17%	308	48%
Rotary, Round Table, Lions and similar men's organisations	384	10%	114	30%
Local community groups (including tenants associations, ratepayers organisations, amenity groups etc.)	915	24%	383	42%
National action groups (CPAG, Shelter, CASE, NCCL etc.)	360	9%	67	19%
Organisations primarily concerned with immigrants	164*	5%	86*	52%

* This figure does not include the results from the South East Thames region where the relevant data are not available. The % is also calculated excluding the South East Thames region.

2.14   MEMBERSHIP OF TRADE UNIONS,
POLITICAL PARTIES AND CHURCHES

	Individuals who are members (N = 3,796)		Individuals holding a position (N = number of members)		Prefer not to state (N = 3,796)	
Trades Unions and Trades Councils	1,113	29%	525	47%	Not asked	
Political parties	2,099	55%	1,073	51%	578	15%
Churches or religious organisations	2,023	53%	Not asked		403	11%

2.15 MEMBERSHIP OF POLITICAL PARTIES

	Total survey (N = 3,796)		Survey: party members only (N = 2,099)	October 1974 Election results England and Wales
Member of a political party:	2,099	55%		
of which:				
Conservative party	696	18%	33%	38%
Labour party	1,133	30%	54%	41%
Liberal party	175	5%	8%	20%
Other party	20	*	1%	1%
Party not stated	75	2%	4%	—
			100%	100%

* Less than one percent.

2.16 PARTY MEMBERSHIP BY NOMINATING GROUPS

	Local authority nominees %	Voluntary organisation nominees %	RHA nominees %
Members of Conservative party	26	10	12
Members of Labour party	48	10	19
Members of Liberal party	6	4	2
None of these*	20	76	66
	100% (N = 1750)	100% (N = 1434)	100% (N = 606)

* These figures include the 20 members of other parties, those who are not members of any party and those for whom no information is known.

2.17 PARTY MEMBERSHIP OF THE SOCIAL CLASS GROUPS

	Professionals and managers		White collar workers		Blue collar workers	
Members of the Conservative party	394	19%	198	19%	40	7%
Members of the Labour party	391	19%	309	30%	359	66%
Members of the Liberal party	110	5%	48	5%	13	2%
None of these*	1,159	56%	474	46%	130	24%
	2,054	100%	1,029	100%	542	100%

* These figures include the 20 members of other parties, those who are not members of any party, and those for whom no information is known.

2.18 LOCAL AUTHORITY MEMBERSHIP AMONG THE NOMINATING GROUPS

	Current Councillor of any local authority		Current Councillor of any local authority except parish councils		
Total survey	1,579	42%	1,473	39%	(N = 3,796)
Local authority nominees	1,444	82%	1,421	81%	(N = 1,750)
Voluntary organisation nominees	84	6%	32	2%	(N = 1,434)
RHA nominees	50	8%	19	3%	(N = 606)
	Past Councillor of any local authority		Past Councillor of any local authority except parish councils		
Total survey	1,543	41%	1,438	38%	(N = 3,796)
Local authority nominees	1,234	70%	1,183	68%	(N = 1,750)
Voluntary organisation nominees	177	12%	135	9%	(N = 1,434)
RHA nominees	129	21%	118	19%	(N = 606)

2.19 **THE NUMBER OF LOCAL AUTHORITY NOMINEES WHO ARE NOT OR HAVE NOT BEEN LOCAL COUNCILLORS**

	Total number of local authority nominees (= N)	LA nominees who are not currently councillors		The number of these who have never been councillors	
East Anglia	72	4	5%	3	4%
Mersey	103	17	16%	10	10%
Northern	131	10	8%	7	5%
North East Thames	120	34	28%	23	19%
North West Thames	143	54	38%	40	28%
North Western	131	28	21%	8	6%
Oxford	68	2	3%	2	3%
South East Thames	135	25	18%	not available	
South West Thames	88	18	20%	14	16%
South Western	109	6	5%	1	1%
Trent	143	28	20%	20	14%
Wales	162	4	2%	1	1%
Wessex	57	2	3%	1	2%
West Midlands	174	44	25%	35	20%
Yorkshire	114	23	20%	13	11%
Total:	1,750	299	17%	—	—
Total excluding South East Thames	1,615	204	13%	178	11%

2.20 NUMBER OF POSITIONS* HELD BY NOMINATING GROUPS

	Total Survey %	Local authority nominees %	Voluntary organisation nominees %	RHA nominees %
None	37	15	61	42
One	39	51	26	33
Two	18	26	9	16
Three	5	7	3	7
Four or more	1	2	1	2
	100% (N = 3796)	100% (N = 1750)	100% (N = 1434)	100% (N = 606)

* These are: magistrates, school governors, co-opted members of local authority committees, members of tribunals or members of consultative councils of nationalised industries.

2.21 POSITIONS HELD BY THE DIFFERENT NOMINATING GROUPS

	Total Survey		Local authority nominees		Voluntary organisation nominees		RHA nominees	
School governors	2,000	53%	1,396	80%	355	25%	247	41%
Magistrates	493	13%	296	17%	102	7%	94	15%
	(N = 3,796)		(N = 1,750)		(N = 1,434)		(N = 606)	

2.22 HEALTH COMMITTEE MEMBERSHIP BY REGIONS

	Membership of a health committee	HMC	RHB	LA health committee	Executive Council	Teaching hospital	Hospital House Committee	Other committee	
	%	%	%	%	%	%	%	%	
East Anglia	38	16	1	20	10	0	8	7	(N = 148)
Mersey	41	10	1	26	9	3	10	8	(N = 229)
Northern	46	21	2	27	8	*	8	8	(N = 315)
North East Thames	35	16	1	22	4	5	10	4	(N = 251)
North West Thames	35	11	1	21	2	4	9	6	(N = 327)
North Western	41	11	1	29	6	*	6	8	(N = 271)
Oxford	41	9	2	24	4	1	12	5	(N = 139)
South East Thames	37	12	2	23	3	2	n.a.	7	(N = 228)
South West Thames	38	11	2	19	2	4	10	6	(N = 185)
South Western	47	20	3	22	7	1	20	10	(N = 230)
Trent	39	15	1	20	7	1	8	6	(N = 315)
Wales	46	12	2	27	4	1	19	7	(N = 364)
Wessex	50	23	2	19	9	1	23	6	(N = 124)
West Midlands	30	11	1	15	5	1	7	6	(N = 361)
Yorkshire	39	19	1	19	8	1	16	4	(N = 249)
Total	39	14	2	22	6	2	11	7	(N = 3,796)

2.23   HEALTH COMMITTEE MEMBERSHIP BY NOMINATING GROUPS

	Local authority nominees		Voluntary organisation nominees		RHA nominees		Total Survey	
No health committee	875	50%	1,113	78%	272	45%	2,264	60%
Hospital Management Committee	200	11%	114	8%	222	37%	537	14%
Regional Hospital Board	20	1%	11	1%	27	4%	59	2%
Local authority health committee	684	39%	84	6%	79	13%	848	22%
Executive Council	125	7%	24	2%	63	10%	212	6%
Teaching hospital	30	2%	7	*	25	4%	63	2%
Hospital House Committee	150	9%	131	9%	117	19%	399	11%
Other Health Committee	109	6%	84	6%	58	10%	251	7%
Not stated	13	1%	11	1%	1	*	25	1%
	125% (N = 1,750)		110% (N = 1,434)		142% (N = 606)		125% (N = 3,796)	

2.24 OCCUPATION (PRESENT AND PAST)

Doctors and dentists	60	2%	occupations in health, social and other public services 42%
Nurses	196	5%	
Ancillary health service staff including those working for local authorities	211	6%	
Civil servants	125	3%	
Social workers	159	4%	
Local government employees excluding those in health and social services	167	4%	
Teachers	280	7%	
Clergymen	136	4%	
Full time workers in voluntary organisations	182	5%	
Any other health or social service related work	64	2%	
Any other occupation	1,884	50%	
Not classified	332	9%	
		100%	
		(N = 3,796)	

2.25 OCCUPATION BY NOMINATING BODY

	Total Survey	Local authorities nominees	Voluntary organisation nominees	RHA nominees
Occupation in health, social and other public services	42% (N = 3,796)	29% (N = 1,750)	56% (N = 1,434)	45% (N = 606)

2.26   DIFFERENCES BETWEEN CHAIRMAN, VICE—CHAIRMAN AND MEMBERS

	Chairman	Vice-Chairman	Members	Total Survey
Total number (= N)	171	143	3482	3796
	%	%	%	%
Male	78	69	55	57
Female	22	31	45	43
Lived in the district for over 15 years	78	67	67	67
Local authority nominees	53	48	46	46
Voluntary organisation nominees	18	31	39	38
RHA nominees	29	21	15	16
Under 44	16	28	28	28
45-54	27	24	30	29
55-64	38	29	28	28
65 +	18	18	14	14
No children under 16	72	64	65	65
Elementary schools	16	17	15	15
Secondary schools	5	7	10	10
Grammar & Public Schools	78	73	73	73
Professional and managerial	58	55	54	54
White collar	26	27	27	27
Blue collar	11	13	15	15
Some further education	49	52	44	44
Some qualifications	82	83	79	79
University degree	31	31	19	20
Working full-time	54	55	51	51
Housewife	5	16	16	16
Retired	22	20	16	17
Occupation in health, social and public services	35	41	42	41
Current councillor excluding parish councillors	47	41	38	39
Magistrate	32	24	12	13
School governor	74	62	51	53
Member of a consultative council	13	10	7	7
Tribunal member	18	15	9	9
Past member of a health committee	73	59	37	39

2.27   **MEMBERSHIP OF SPECIAL CARE GROUPS BY NOMINATING GROUPS**

	Local authority nominees		Voluntary organisation nominees		RHA nominees			Total Survey (N = 3,796)
Groups concerned with:								
Mentally handicapped	188	38%	248	51%	53	11%	100% (N = 490)	13%
Mental health	106	28%	207	55%	60	16%	100% (N = 373)	10%
Physically disabled	210	35%	317	53%	72	12%	100% (N = 600)	16%
Elderly	471	50%	384	41%	87	9%	100% (N = 942)	25%
Children and maternity	126	34%	193	52%	52	14%	100% (N = 371)	10%

2.28   **DISTRIBUTION OF VOLUNTARY ORGANISATION MEMBERSHIP BY NOMINATING GROUPS**

	Member of:-						
	No organisations %	One %	Two %	Three %	Four %	Over Four %	
Local authority nominees	24	26	20	13	8	9	(N = 1750) 100%
Voluntary organisation nominees	3	24	25	21	12	13	(N = 1434) 100%
RHA nominees	16	25	26	17	9	7	(N = 606) 100%

2.29 MEMBERSHIP OF CIVIC AND COMMUNITY GROUPS BY NOMINATING GROUPS

	Local authority nominees	Voluntary organisation nominees	RHA nominees		Total survey (N = 3796)
Women's organisations	229 36%	316 49%	100 15%	(N = 645) 100%	17%
Men's organisations	157 41%	144 38%	82 21%	(N = 384) 100%	10%
Local community groups	494 54%	289 32%	131 14%	(N = 915) 100%	24%
National action groups	152 42%	155 43%	53 15%	(N = 360) 100%	9%
Immigrant organisations	81 49%	58 35%	25 15%	(N = 164) 100%	5%
Trade Unions	740 66%	217 19%	156 14%	(N = 1113) 100%	29%
Churches	901 44%	780 39%	338 17%	(N = 2023) 100%	53%

2.30   VARIATIONS BETWEEN THE DIFFERENT NOMINATING GROUPS

	Local authority nominees	Voluntary organisation nominees	RHA nominees	Total survey
	%	%	%	%
Professional and managerial	42	64	65	54
White collar	30	26	22	27
Blue collar	23	6	9	15
Male	67	43	60	57
Female	33	56	40	43
Grammer or public schools	64	81	79	73
Some full-time further education	39	48	54	45
Some qualifications	66	82	80	74
University degree	15	22	29	20
Working full-time	55	46	54	51
Working part-time	9	13	10	11
Unpaid work	6	16	8	10
Housewife	13	19	15	16
Retired	18	15	16	17
Under 34	10	9	7	9
35-44	17	19	18	18
45-54	28	31	29	29
55-64	26	29	32	28
65 +	17	11	14	14
	(N = 1750)	(N = 1434)	(N = 606)	(N = 3796)

3

Views
and verdicts

When Community Health Councils were first set up, two contradictory fears were expressed. On the one hand, there was apprehension within the National Health Service — among administrators, doctors, nurses and other professionals — that these strange new animals would add to the problems of reorganisation: that they would magnify and exacerbate individual complaints and introduce the grit of public controversy into the administrative machinery of the service. On the other hand, there was the opposing fear within the consumer lobby — among what might be called professional consumers — that CHCs would be too deferential towards the health service authorities and adopt the recessive style of the consultative committees attached to the nationalised industries[1]. Public policy, as noted in the first chapter, was largely hammered out in a series of compromises between those who were anxious to avoid creating institutionalised trouble-makers and those who were equally determined to ensure that the CHCs should be encouraged to be both independent and outspoken — or, to make this distinction another way, between those who thought that the first loyalty of CHC members ought to be to the National Health Service and those who believed that their only responsibility was to voice the views of the consumer.

But how do CHC members themselves see their role? Do they, in fact, conform to either of the stereotypes implicit in the debates about setting up CHCs? To what extent are they (to caricature the argument) either deferential or **antaganistic**? Do they have views which are either sympathetic or hostile to the NHS? In this chapter, we discuss our survey information bearing, directly or indirectly, on such questions. Before doing so, it may be helpful to set out what the data collected can and cannot tell us. Most crucially our survey provides a snap-shot at one point in time. The CHC members were asked to give their views — on a whole variety of issues — soon after first taking office. Some of them even complained that they had not been given a chance to give an educated reaction to our questionnaire in the light of experience: but, of course, the intention was to look at the human raw material coming into the machine, not at the transformations operated on that raw material by contact with the NHS. The advantage of this approach is that it provides information about the beliefs and prejudices of the recruits; the disadvantage is that it tells us nothing about their views after experience of service on CHCs and exposure to the problems of the NHS. Our data throughout is about the opinions of CHCs members, not about the underlying attitudes — and it is generally recognised that opinions, in contrast to attitudes, are not necessarily stable or deep-rooted [2].

In analysing the data, it would obviously have been interesting to look at variations between individual CHCs. But, once again, a response rate which is high enough to allow statements to be made about the national total — and regional differences within it — does not necessarily allow a comparison of individual CHCs. Further, in contrast to the previous chapter, we use regional comparisons more sparingly and only where there appears to be a particular and positive reason for thinking that there might be a geographical dimension to variations in the opinions expressed by CHC members: otherwise, given the heterogeneity of the regions, it seems more sensible to assume that variations reflect differences in the composition of the membership rather than a specific regional factor, and we concentrate in our analysis on exploring whether different types of CHC members also bring different views to their job.

The data therefore permits us to examine the policy issues raised in the previous chapter from a new perspective: it allows us to ask to what extent social class and the other characteristics of CHC members affect their perception of their own role and their assessments of the NHS. In short: does who they are make any difference to what they think about what they ought to be doing?

What the CHC should be doing

Given the ambiguities inherent in the political and administrative language used to describe the role of CHCs, there seemed to be every reason to ask the members themselves how they saw their role. In our pilot survey of CHC members in the South East Thames region, we asked them to describe in their own words what they saw as the "main job" of the CHCs. Their answers, which were subsequently used in the design of our questionnaire for the main survey, fell broadly into three categories[3]. There were those who saw themselves representing the views of the community to those running the health service: the conventional view, echoing the official circulars and speeches which had provided the overture to the setting-up of CHCs. Then there were those who saw themselves as middle-men, between the consumers and the management, acting as a two-way channel of information. Lastly, and perhaps most surprisingly, there were a few CHC members who saw themselves as the representatives of the NHS to the consumers, creating more understanding for the problems of the service.

In our national survey, the "representatives" are in a majority among CHC members: almost two-thirds give first priority to the CHC's role as being "to represent the community's interest in the health service to those responsible for the management" (Table 3.1). The consumer diplomats who see CHCs as a channel between the NHS and the community, mediating between the two, are a significant minority, at one-third of all CHC members. But the management apologists, who put first emphasis on creating understanding for the NHS, turn out to be a very rare — almost extinct — species. Interestingly, even when they were given an opportunity to give less emphatic support for this view, in naming their second priority, only 15% of CHC members chose to do so.

In this, the method of nomination makes little difference (Table 3.2). Voluntary organisation nominees are just a shade more likely to see themselves as consumer diplomats than local authority nominees, with the RHA nominees coming in between. This is perhaps predictable, since local authority members — particularly if they are elected councillors — may well have a generalised image of themselves as representatives, irrespective of the precise institutional context. More surprising, because both less predictable and more emphatic, are the differences related to the age of CHC councillors. As these grow older, so they are more likely to see themselves as consumer diplomats. Only a quarter of those under 35 see themselves in this role, as against one-third of those between 35 and 55 and two-fifths of those over 55. And, consistent with this, those over 55 are four times more likely to think of themselves as management apologists than those under 35.

To supplement the questions about the general role of the CHC, members were next asked to rank their order of priorities from a list of six specific functions. This list was compiled partly on the basis of the replies given to an open-ended question in the pilot survey — which, for example, revealed an unexpected interest in improving conditions for NHS staff — and partly on the DHSS's catalogue of "matters to which Community Health Councils might wish to direct their attention". Overwhelmingly CHC members give, as their first priority, one of the job-descriptions taken from the DHSS's catalogue: the most important function of the CHC — according to 69% of them — is "to review the standards of local services and future plans" (Tables 3.3 and 14A).

This collective view suggests that the policy makers were successful in impressing on CHC members that they should play a constructively helpful rather than critically destructive role in the NHS. But it also indicates potential for stress among CHC members when it comes to translating general aspirations and official rhetoric about what they should be doing into the small-change of every-day behaviour, since it is not altogether easy to reconcile the emphasis on representation noted above and the more managerial stance implicit in the emphasis on reviewing standards and plans.

In contrast to this overwhelming emphasis on reviewing plans and assessing services — a function which is so generously wide and vague that it can arguably embrace almost anything a CHC might wish to do — there is much less support for the other, more specific items on the list. Second in the mean rank ordering [4], but a long way behind, comes "to advise and publicise to the man in the street the facilities available", followed by "to be concerned about the way waiting lists and appointment systems are organised". Both these obtain only 11% of the first preferences. The fact that so few CHC members feel passionately about waiting lists is, perhaps, surprising, given that this is a perennially sensitive issue. But it is consistent with the low priority attached to assisting people to put their complaints. This, again, suggests that politically salient issues are not necessarily those which most excite the interests of CHC members. Only three per cent of them give their first vote to this function; the same proportion assign first priority to ensuring good working conditions for NHS staff — although the latter does come lower in the mean rank order.

This lack of emphasis on the complaints-processing function is open to two, quite different interpretations. It may mean that CHC members spontaneously attach greater importance to dealing with general planning issues than with specific, individual cases. Alternatively, it may simply reflect their dutiful reproduction of the official doctrine that they should think positively rather than engaging in such negative activities as handling grievances. To the extent that the latter explanation holds, so the low priority attached to complaints-processing may be a poor predictor of behaviour. An indication of the possible gap between opinions and actions is given by the fact that only two per cent of CHC members give concern about quality of food and amenities for hospital patients as their first priority, and that this function is fifth in the overall ranking. Yet, in practice, CHCs have shown a great deal of concern about the housekeeping aspects of the health service: this emerges quite clearly from the first set of annual reports, analysed in the next chapter.

In all this, there is a danger that aggregating the data from all our CHC members may imply a spurious homogeneity of views. For instance, it might not be unreasonable to expect views about functions to vary according to the source of nomination — particularly since, as seen already, these groups bring rather difference experiences to their CHC work. In fact, such variations are slight (Table 3.4). All groups have the same overall rank orderings, although there are differences of emphasis within them. Voluntary organisation and RHA nominees are somewhat more likely to support reviewing standards and planning than local authority members; in turn, local authority nominees attach rather more priority to waiting lists, assisting with complaints and ensuring good working conditions for NHS staff than the other two groups.

One reason for these differences of emphasis could lie in the social class composition of the three sets of nominees[5]. And, in the event, analysing the priorities given to different CHC functions by social class does show quite pronounced variations. Most conspicuously, the higher the social class, the more concern is shown about reviewing standards and planning; conversely, but less emphatically, the blue-collar CHC members attach more importance to waiting lists and ensuring good working conditions for NHS staff than do either white-collar workers or professionals and managers. To some extent this may reflect the occupational background of the latter two categories. As noted earlier, these are disproportionately concentrated in the social and public services, and it would therefore not be surprising if they took a somewhat "managerial" approach to the problem of consumer representation in the NHS. This explanation is consistent with the fact that those in this broad occupational classification tend to be more concerned about standards and planning than the rest of CHC councillors.

Overall, then, the evidence would suggest that different methods of recruitment — to the degree that they bring to representative bodies a greater spread of social interests — do help also to ensure a wider spectrum of views than might otherwise be the case. This said, it is important to stress that while social class variations do exist, they are differences in shading, not differences in kind. It is just as important to note that *all* social classes give first priority to the planning function as to register the fact that there are slight variations between them. In the evidence reviewed so far there is no sign that the hierarchy of values differs either by social class or by nominating bodies, although there may be variations in the degrees of emphasis.

Assessing the services

So far the survey results suggest that the members recruited to the CHCs did not, on taking on their job, view their functions in an aggressively critical way. They seem to identify almost as much with the problems of those running the service as with the problems of the consumer. But how do they view the quality of the services actually provided? To find out, we asked CHCs to give their rating — good, adequate or unsatisfactory — of the health services in their district: ratings which, it must be stressed again, reflect their perceptions as members of the public rather than as informed councillors — since they had not yet had time to educate themselves about the state of the services in their new role.

Overwhelmingly CHC members consider the services to be either good or adequate: a third taking the former view and a half expressing the latter opinion (Table 3.5). Less than a fifth think that the services are unsatisfactory. This would suggest that if, over the years, the CHCs collectively become critical of the NHS, it will be because of what they learn about the service from the inside rather than because of any prejudices or biases they brought to their job in the first place.

In expressing satisfaction with the NHS, if with varying degrees of enthusiasm, CHC members accurately mirror the views of the population at large. In the autumn of 1974, for example, NOP asked a sample of the public about their views on the NHS [6] and, allowing for the difference in the wording of the questions, the results were virtually identical with those from our survey. What is more, the views of the public about the NHS are astonishingly stable and and unaffected by what is happening in the service. In January 1976 when NOP again inquired into opinions about the health service — a period when there was much talk about the impending collapse of the NHS because of consultant discontent, union troubles and inadequate finance — there was no sign of any diminution in satisfaction or increase in dissatisfaction. Further, much the same picture of consumer satisfaction is conveyed by other surveys: for example, that conducted on behalf of the Royal Commission on the Constitution[7]. Possibly, consumers may be much more prepared to settle for the *status quo* than the service providers.

One explanation for the high degree of satisfaction could be low expectations. The figures, it may be argued, tell us nothing about whether or not there is anything wrong with the NHS but only about the low standards or deferential attitudes of the consuming public. If that were the case, it would be reasonable to expect satisfaction with the NHS to vary with social class: the higher the social class, it could be argued, the more dissatisfied people are likely to be since they are more likely to be knowledgeable about the scope for improvement[8]. In fact, there is no real evidence of this among CHC members (Table 3.6). Rather fewer of the professionals and managers than of the blue-collar workers regard their local services as good (30% as against 33%); rather more of the latter than of the former declare them to be unsatisfactory (21% as against 16%). Once again, this is consistent with the findings of the NOP poll, which showed there to be no difference in satisfaction by social class.

If satisfaction with the NHS is not linked to social class, some of the other characteristics of CHC members could well be relevant. For example, women use the NHS in different ways from men, and this might be reflected in their views. But the evidence is ambiguous. A higher proportion of men than women consider the service unsatisfactory — 20% as against 15% — though exactly the same proportion think it is good. More interestingly assessments vary sharply by age. The older CHC members are, the more satisfied they profess themselves to be with the NHS. Those under 35 are three times less likely to think the service good than those over 55, and three times more likely to think it unsatisfactory. In this respect, the CHC members appear to be atypical of the population at large since other surveys suggest that satisfaction does not vary perceptibly with age; this might suggest that the younger recruits to public positions are, perhaps, distinguished by their more critical attitudes — and that it is a commitment to changing things which brings them onto CHCs, and similar bodies, in the first place. The age effect does not appear to be explained by the social class composition of the various groups (Table 15A). The under 35s have the highest proportion of professionals and managers who, as seen already, are the least dissatisfied.

In all this, the opinions of the CHC members about their local services seem to reflect some fairly stable views, and are more than a set of random, off-the-cuff reactions to an importunate questionnaire. This is shown by the consistency of the answers to various questions. The relationship between the views about the role of the CHC (see above) and the assessments of the service is precisely what would be expected (Table 3.7). Those who believe that the role of the CHC ought to be to create understanding for the problems of the NHS — whom we have christened, somewhat unkindly, management apologists — are much more likely to rate the service good, and much less prone to be dissatisfied, than those who think that the role of the CHC is to put the views of the community to the administrators. And the consumer diplomats — those who see the CHCs acting as a channel between the community and the NHS — neatly fall in between the other two groups in their assessment of local services: they are more likely to think the service good and less likely to be dissatisfied than the representatives.

Apart from the personal characteristics of the CHC members, their previous experience might also colour their views. For example, those nominated by voluntary organisations might be expected to be more critical — assuming that critical views reflect past experience of the short-comings of the NHS. In fact, however, this does not turn out to be the case: there is little to choose between the assessment of local authority and voluntary organisation nominees. If anything, the former are a shade more critical. Those nominated by the RHAs tend to be marginally more satisfied than the rest. One reason for this could be that the RHA nominees have, as already noted, greater previous experience of health authority membership. Such experience seems to breed a more favourable assessment of the NHS: 38% of those who have served on health authorities (and thus perhaps gained an opportunity to see the problems from the insider's point of view) assess the local NHS provision as good, as against only 27% for the other CHC members.

In contrast to the views on the role and functions of CHCs, there is every reason to anticipate geographical variations in the assessment of services since the quality and level of the NHS provision is far from uniform[9]. And this turns out to be the case (Tables 3.8 and 16A). the proportion of those who think the local service is good ranges from 24% in the North East Thames to 42% in the South Western region; the proportion of those who consider the local service unsatisfactory ranges from seven per cent in Wessex and the Northern to 27% in the North East Thames and the Trent regions.

One possible explanation might be that these variations reflect differences in the personal characteristics of CHC members. The most important of these, in respect of the assessment of services is, as we have just seen, the age of members. And, in the event the dissatisfied regions tend to be younger regions. But, given the small numbers involved, this factor can only explain some of the regional differences. As well as searching for subjective differences in the way health services are perceived, it therefore seems sensible to look also at the objective differences in the health services themselves. If people are dissatisfied with the local health services, the most obvious explanation could be that these services are inadequate — and *vice versa.*

The difficulty of testing whether or not there is a relationship between the assessments made and the adequacy of the service provided stems from the absence of any agreed criteria for judging quality in the provision of health care. For lack of anything better, there is a tendency to infer quality from expenditure — and to assume that the more money is spent, the better services will be. This, at any rate, is the assumption on which public policy has been built: the current policy of the DHSS is to iron out inequalities in regional *per capita* spending and to move towards a situation where, allowing for differences in population structure, all regions will be spending the same amount [10]. Equal expenditure is thus taken to imply equal treatment in the double sense of social fairness and of access to medical care.

Unfortunately, to judge by the views of the CHC members, equal expenditure does not appear to lead to equal satisfaction. In terms of expenditure per head of population, for example, Oxford and Wessex are identical. But the former is a critical region, while the latter is a satisfied one. Comparing the rankings of the regions for, first, expenditure and, second, the proportion of CHC members who consider their local services "good", shows little correspondence between the two sets of figures. The Trent region is consistent in being both the poorest and in having a high level of dissatisfaction. But the metropolitan regions combine top-ranking for expenditure and low-ranking for satisfaction. While there are some indications that the more rural regions tend to be happier about their local health service — witness Wessex, once again, and East Anglia — this does not account so neatly for the high degree of satisfaction in the Northern and Yorkshire regions. In contrast, there is a fairly solid belt of dissatisfaction in the urban areas which stretch from London, through the Midlands, to Manchester.

As always, the regions are themselves heterogeneous. And, as always, the problem of response rate makes it very difficult to analyse differences within regions — or to relate the views of individual CHCs to specific local circumstances(11). For example, the most critical CHC in the satisfied South Western region has a higher proportion of members who consider the service unsatisfactory than the most critical CHC in the dissatisfied South West Thames — 29% as against 22%. And even in the North East Thames, which has the smallest proportion of CHC members of any region who think that their local service is good, there are oases of contentment: in South Camden, none of the respondents to the survey thought the service unsatisfactory.

It is, unfortunately, impossible — on the evidence available to us — to find any consistent patterns in these variations. About the only firm conclusion that emerges is that isolation appears to breed satisfaction: both the Isles of Scilly and Anglesey emerge as satisfied communities, with hardly any criticism of the local health service. Taking the other extreme — those CHCs where not a single respondent thought that the local service was good — there are East Cumbria, Wigan and North Surrey. It is a curious list, and it seems that the explanation for a common factor must be sought in local conditions and in local perceptions of adequacy. Otherwise it is difficult to see what northern industrial workers and London commuters have in common.

In turn, it would be interesting to be able to relate the patterns of judgment about the adequacy of local services to the patterns of resource distribution in the NHS. Does a high level of resources lead to a high level of satisfaction? In the regions, there was little evidence of any such link. But in the CHC districts, it would be reasonable to anticipate a more direct relationship. Unfortunately information about expenditure levels directly relevant to CHCs is only available for single-district Areas. And the 14 single-district Areas where the CHC response rate was over 60% (and where the "can't say" category was 25% or less) present a mixed picture. In four out of the five poorest districts there is an excess of CHC members dissatisfied with the local services over those who think that these are good. So, at the extreme, poverty of resources may be linked to dissatisfaction. But, thereafter, it is difficult to see any sort of relationship between spending and the assessment of services on the basis of our admittedly sketchy and inadequate information (Table 3.9).

No conclusions for policy can be drawn on the basis of evidence drawn from a handful of individual CHCs. But since the regional analysis also indicated a lack of correspondence between assessment of services and the level of expenditure, our survey does suggest that the case for re-distributing resources to the less well-to-do regions rests primarily on political and professional notions of fairness and social justice. It does not appear to reflect accurately, consumer views (as represented by CHC members) and may not even lead to consumer gratitude. To sum up the evidence on this point, in five out of the seven regions which are to have their expenditure levels cut under the redistribution formula the CHC members are also above-average for dissatisfaction, while in three out of the seven which will gain they are above-average for satisfaction. This could indicate that consumer assessment of services — in as far as it is measured by the views of the CHC members — depends much more on the local organisation of the delivery of services than on the level of expenditure, and perhaps also on the way resources are apportioned in any particular place between different sectors of the NHS. The next section therefore examines the views of the CHC members about specific services, either operated by the NHS or relevant to it.

Problems and priorities

Any general assessment of a service as complex and many-sided as the NHS is bound to be an exercise in balancing various judgments. To complement the question about the views of CHC members on the overall standards of health care provision in their district, we provided them with a list of individual services and asked them whether they presented any particular problems and, if so, to indicate the degree of severity. This list included two services only partly operated by the NHS, domiciliary care and transport, since our pilot survey had shown that these were areas of concern to CHC members. This not only allows us to look in more detail at the specific worries of CHC members — the bias of their appreciation systems (13) on taking office — but also to examine more closely the texture of dissatisfaction by region: to see whether the shoe is felt to pinch in the same spot everywhere.

In the event, a distinct pattern emerges from the perceptions of CHC members about problems in specific services (Table 3.10). By far the highest proportion, almost two-fifths of those giving a positive answer, think that the long stay hospitals present an urgent problem to their CHC: this is very much in line with what might be called conventional wisdom. But, rather surprisingly, it is transport and domiciliary care — rather than any of the services exclusively provided by the NHS — which come next in the hierarchy of problem areas: almost one-third and just under a quarter, respectively, of CHC members see these as presenting urgent problems in their district. Just over a fifth of CHC members perceive urgent problems in the general hospital services. Paradoxically the perception of problems becomes less urgent as the frequency of use increases. For most people, contact with the NHS is — for most of the time — contact with their family doctor: it is the GP who deals with nine out of ten episodes of illness. But less than a tenth of CHC members see any urgent problems in this sector. Even allowing for the fact that 64% did perceive some problems — much the same percentage as for other services mentioned so far — this suggests that the family practitioner service is regarded as working more satisfactorily than either the hospital services or the supporting services in the community. A lower proportion still of CHC members are worried about the pharmaceutical services — although self-treatment, with the help of the chemist, is even more frequent than consulting the GP [14].

In interpreting these figures, there is special need for care. A far higher proportion of CHC members felt unable to answer the question about specific problems than any of the other items in our questionnaire. So the conclusions about the problem-orientation of CHC members refers only to those who felt confident or informed enough to give their views. The "can't say" category is, however, interesting in its own right: it may indicate the varying degrees to which different services impinge on the public consciousness. For instance, the proportion of non-respondents was highest for the pharmaceutical services which are also perceived to offer the fewest urgent problems. Similarly, if somewhat less predictably, the dental services drew both a low response rate and a low urgency rating.

Views on specific services can reasonably be expected to be coloured by the experiences of individual CHC members, and to a limited extent this turns out to be the case (Table 3.11). Some are related to sex: women tend to see more urgent problems than men in four of the seven services on the list — the main exceptions being general hospital and general practitioner services. Again, there are differences by nominating body. The problem perceptions of voluntary organisation nominees are remarkably similar to those of the women CHC members: they are generally more critical than either the local authority or RHA nominees — with the exception, once again, of general hospital and general practitioner services.

These patterns are capable of two — not necessarily mutually exclusive —explanations. There are, as noted earlier, a higher proportion of women among voluntary organisation nominees than in either of the other two categories. So it could be that it is membership of voluntary organisations — in particular those concerned with the special care groups — which makes women more aware of the shortcomings of the long-stay hospitals and domiciliary services. Alternatively, the identity of view could reflect the fact that it is women who do the caring and thus become sensitive to the failings of the caring services (while men are more concerned about the curing services).

The other relevant characteristic in helping to shape views about specific services once again turns out to be the age of the CHC member. Not only are younger CHC members more critical in their general assessment of their local NHS service, but they are also more likely to perceive urgent problems in specific areas of provision. In six out of the seven services on the list, there is a steady increase in the perception of urgent problems as age falls. The pattern is so consistent as to suggest that our questions are tapping an underlying difference in attitude. The CHC members under 35 are, it appears, less deferential and more critical than the others. Certainly age seems more important than social class where the differences are less pronounced but where blue-collar workers (predictably, given that these are disproportionately male and nominated by local authorities) tend to be slightly more critical of general hospital and family practitioner services than either professionals and managers or white-collar workers.

Turning to the geographical variations, it is difficult to be sure about the extent to which these reflect specific regional health service factors as distinct from differences in the composition of the membership. But the regional variations (Table 3.12) are larger than might have been expected from the differences in composition — the number of under 35s is small everywhere — and not always in the direction that would have been predicted from looking at the characteristics of the CHC members. Wales is well above-average for the proportion of men among its CHC members yet below average in the percentage perceiving any urgent problems in general hospital and general practitioner services.

There is a further problem in trying to interpret regional variations. These could reflect either differences in the services themselves or differences in expectations, attitudes and perceptions. After all, there might well be a regional social culture in the sense of a shared set of values about what to expect from public services. On this point, our evidence does not permit any definite conclusions: particularly since the two explanations are not necessarily contradictory, and differences based on objective factors might well be refracted — to a lesser or greater degree — through the lens of local preconceptions about standards.

This said, the regional variations are so large that it would require a very contrasted pattern of social cultures and perceptions to explain them.

For domiciliary services, the proportion of those reporting urgent problems ranges from 17% to 33%; for transport, it is 16% to 42%; for pharmaceutical services, it is from one per cent to 15%; for long-stay hospitals, it is from 29% to 48%; for dental services, it is from seven to 36%; for general practice, it is from one per cent to 15%. Moreover, if the explanation of the variations is to be found in the general stance of CHC members, then it would be reasonable to expect them to be internally consistent: that is, to be either critical or appreciative of *all* services. In fact, CHC members appear to discriminate, to some extent at least, between services and not just to bestow a blanket blessing or condemnation. Oxford, for example, is consistent in being fairly, but not extremely, critical of all services. East Anglia, in contrast, perceives fewer urgent problems than any other regions in its long-stay hospitals but more than any other region in the dental and transport services. The South Western region is somewhat different, yet again, in that it is at the national average in its perception of problems in long-stay hospitals and general hospital services but is exceptionally satisfied with the dental and general practitioner services.

This last point suggests an intriguing possibility: that it is the perception of the adequacy or otherwise of the general practitioner services which shapes the overall appreciation of the service provided by the NHS. This is not an unreasonable supposition given that, as already pointed out, for most of the time health service consumers never get beyond their family practitioner in their contacts with the NHS. And, indeed, a comparison of the rankings of the regions in terms of their general assessment of their local health service (see Table 3.8) and those of the regions in terms of their perceptions of urgent problems in general practice, shows a considerable correspondence. The regions which see the least problems in general practice also tend to show the highest degree of satisfaction in their overall view of the NHS, and *vice versa*. Given the earlier finding that there is only a tenuous and uncertain relationship between satisfaction and expenditure per head, this would suggest that to the extent that it is the aim of public expenditure to maximise public satisfaction, then Governments should be increasing spending on the primary care sector but not on the rest of the NHS — which is, in effect, what is happening [15].

So far the analysis has dealt only with the broad-brush views of CHC members about large sectors in the NHS and related services. It has not attempted to explore their predispositions in terms of specific care groups: or to establish their views about what they think ought to be done, for whom. Yet clearly such predispositions are important and, moreover, planning in the NHS is increasingly coming to mean resource allocation for particular groups of people, as distinct from the traditional emphasis on institutions and sectors of health care. Accordingly, we asked CHC members to rank their personal priorities in a list of eight care groups. These included both those care groups which are conventionally picked out for special attention — like the mentally handicapped and ill, the physically handicapped and the elderly, mothers and children — and two larger categories: what we described as acutely ill patients and ordinary patients. By the former, we meant those in urgent requirement of care; by the latter we meant those who needed no more than routine attention. But, obviously, the distinction between what is "acute", or urgent, and what is "ordinary", or routine, is partly subjective, and the answers to these two questions must be interpreted with this reservation in mind. Taken together these two questions provide a rough-and-ready indication of the extent to which CHC members give priority to services for those NHS consumers who do not fall into the special care categories.

In the event, the priorities of the CHC members are those which might be expected from a set of people who had listened to the pronouncement of Ministers about the deficiencies of the NHS's chronic care sector and who had paid heed to stories of neglect or worse which emerged from a series of inquiries into conditions in long-stay institutions. Their priorities (Tables 3.13 and 17A) echo the accepted and acceptable views about the NHS: the mentally ill, the elderly and the mentally handicapped emerge as the most favoured groups in that they are given the highest mean rankings. In this, the CHC members appear to agree with the Government's policies as set out in the 1976 Consultative Document [16]. The Government's aims are slightly different in putting most emphasis on the elderly and the mentally handicapped, rather than on the mentally ill; but CHC members and the DHSS are at one, seemingly, in giving a low ranking to acute and general hospital services and the hospital maternity services. The consensus is all the more remarkable in that our survey was completed months before the DHSS issued its consultative document.

Whether this consensus would survive the strains of actually implementing the Government's priorities is less clear. The views of CHC members suggest that many of them might not be prepared to accept the full implications of giving low priority to the general and acute hospital services (which would mean, in effect *cutting* some of these in areas of high provision). For concentrating on the mean rank of the priorities given to particular groups distracts attention from the existence of an intense and far from insignificant minority of CHC members who put the claims of the ordinary NHS consumer (whether requiring acute or routine care) before those of the special care categories. Just over a fifth give first priority to the acutely ill patient and just over a tenth give first priority to ordinary patients: the former get more first priority votes than any other group, if only by a hair's breadth. So it cannot be assumed, on the basis of the evidence of our survey, that CHC members as a whole would accept a set of priorities which, while improving conditions for the elderly or the mentally ill, implied a decline or standstill in standards for other patients. Only in the case of maternity services does there appear to be a complete fit between the Government's policy to cut down their resource allocation and the priorities of CHC members.

CHC members are remarkably homogeneous in their priorities. There are few differences — whether by social class or nominating body — and, where they exist, they are small (Table 3.14). Local authority nominees, for example, appear to attach slightly greater priority to acutely ill patients than voluntary organisation members in both their mean rankings and the proportion making this group their first priority. Again, while the RHA nominees, in contrast to both the other groups, give first priority in their rankings to the elderly rather than to the mentally ill the differences are not pronounced. Social class variations are also slight and are worth remarking on chiefly because they confirm what appears to be an emerging and consistent pattern. The priority given to the acutely ill increases as social class falls, consistent with the earlier evidence about the perception of problems in particular services.

But in one respect it would be reasonable to expect a strong link between the background of members and their priorities. Since the system of choosing CHC members is designed to ensure the presence of members with links to voluntary organisations concerned with special care groups, it might be assumed that such loyalties would be reflected in the priorities. And this is, indeed, the case (Table 3.15) — taking the voluntary organisation links of all CHC members, whether or not they were actually nominated by a particular care group constituency. Those who are members of voluntary organisations concerned with the mentally ill and handicapped, the physically handicapped and the elderly all give a higher priority to their own special care group than CHC councillors as a whole. Only those linked with children and maternity services do not show such a predeliction. To this extent, then, CHC members do see themselves as having a special responsibility for particular groups as distinct from playing a neutral role in a collective team. They are, clearly, committed to fighting for their own good cause. However, it is neither a blind nor an unquestioning commitment, and it does not preclude an awareness of the needs of other groups. Those concerned with the mentally handicapped give the most priority to their own group, but even here only a third of them give it first ranking. Those concerned with the elderly and the physically handicapped, while giving above average priority to their own groups, actually give marginally more first ranking choices to the acutely ill. So it seems that the priorities of the CHC members are influenced — but not automatically determined — by their background experience in voluntary organisations. Given this, it is not surprising to find that there is no neat fit between the regional distribution of voluntary organisation membership and the regional pattern of priorities (Table 18A). For example, although the Northern region is conspicuous for the under-representation of voluntary organisations concerned with mental health, CHC councillors there give this group rather higher priority — in the mean ranking — than the average for the country as a whole.

To describe the predispositions of CHC members, as we have been doing here, is not to try to predict how they will behave in practice. We do not know to what extent their opinions represent hopeful aspirations rather than entrenched commitments; nor can we begin to tell how their priorities will be modified when they come into conflict with each other. In the next chapter we therefore turn to examining the activities of CHC members in their first year of office.

1 For an account of these, see Second Report from the Select Committee on Nationalised Industries Session 1970-71. *Relations with the public* HMSO 1971, HC.514.

2 A useful introduction to the literature on this subject is Robert E. Lane and David O. Sears *Public Opinion* Prentice-Hall 1964. Also the various papers in Marie Jahoda and Neil Warren (eds.) *Attitudes* Penguin Books 1966.

3 Since the CHC members in the South East Thames were asked open-ended, not structured, questions. their replies could not be incorporated into the rest of the data. In what follows, therefore, the South East Thames is excluded from both the statistics and from the discussion.

4 For each item in the question, a mean rank order was calculated. This was computed on the basis that first priority $= 1$, second priority $= 2$ and so on.

5 Some evidence that policy interests and biases may be linked to social class is given in Barry Hindess *The decline of working class politics* Paladin 1971. See also Rudolf Klein 'The case for elitism: public opinion and public policy' *Political Quarterly* Oct./Dec. 1974.

6 NOP Political Bulletin No.129, September 1974. The 1976 survey is reported in NOP Political, Social, Economic Review No.6 April 1976. In addition, NOP made available to us some additional, unpublished tables; we are most grateful for this help.

7 Commission on the Constitution. Research Papers No.7 *Devolution and other aspects of Government: an attitude survey* HMSO 1973. See Table 23, which shows that 52% of those interviewed thought that the hospital service was "very good" — a much higher rate of satisfaction than recorded for the other services listed.

8 This is consistent with the findings of Ann Cartwright *Patients and their doctors* Routledge & Kegan Paul 1967. See pages 208 to 209 for the evidence that, on some issues at least, professional people are more demanding than unskilled workers.

9 Martin Buxton and Rudolf Klein 'Distribution of hospital provision: policy themes and resource variations' *British Medical Journal* 8 February 1975.

10 *First interim report of the resource allocation Working Party: allocations to regions in 1976/77* DHSS 1975. For a commentary on Government policy, based on this report, see Martin Buxton *Redistributing health resources: scope, criteria and costs*, Paper given at the Regional Studies Association, 17 March 1976.

11 Once again only those CHCs with a response rate over 60% have been included in the analysis.

12 J.H. Rickard 'Per capita expenditure of the English area health authorities' *British Medical Journal* 31 January 1976. This provides information for all AHAs in England, but of course only the data for the single-district areas among them can be related directly to individual CHCs.

13 The phrase is borrowed from Sir Geoffrey Vickers *The Art of Judgment* Chapman & Hall 1965.

14 W.J.H. Butterfield 'Changing medical needs' in Department of Health and Social Security *National Health Service Twentieth Anniversary Conference Report* HMSO 1968.

15 *Public Expenditure to 1979-80* HMSO 1976. Cmnd.6393.

16 Department of Health and Social Security *Priorities for Health and Personal Social Services in England: A Consultative Document* HMSO 1976.

3.1   THE ROLE OF THE CHC

	First priority %	Second priority %	Third priority %		Not stated (N = 3,508)
"The CHC's job is to represent the community's interest in the health service to those responsible for the management".	63	28	10	100% (N = 3,287)	6% 221
"The CHCs are essentially a channel through which the health authorities and the public can learn of each other's needs and difficulties".	35	57	8	100% (N = 3,285)	6% 223
"The CHC's job is to create understanding among consumers of the problems of the NHS and its staff".	3	15	82	100% (N = 3,273)	7% 235

3.2   DIFFERENCES IN THE PERCEIVED ROLE OF THE CHC

Taking the first priority only

	'Represent' %	'Channel' %	'Understand' %	*
Total sample	63	35	3	(N = 3287) 100%
Local authority nominees	64	32	4	(N = 1510) 100%
Voluntary organisation nominees	60	38	2	(N = 1259) 100%
RHA nominees	63	36	1	(N = 529) 100%
Age under 35	74	25	1	(N = 301) 100%
35-54	65	33	2	(N = 1600) 100%
55 +	56	40	4	(N = 1379) 100%

* The differences between (N) in this column and the survey totals are accounted for by the non-respondents.

3.3   THE FUNCTION OF THE CHC

	Distribution of first priority ranking %	Mean rank
Review standards	69	1.68
Publicise facilities	11	3.12
Waiting lists	11	3.30
Assisting with complaints	3	4.03
Quality of food etc.	2	4.39
Good staff working conditions	3	4.45

The first priority was ranked (1).

3.4 DIFFERING PERCEPTIONS OF THE FUNCTION OF THE CHC

		Review Standards	Publicise facilities	Waiting lists	Assisting with Complaints	Quality of food	Good staff working conditions
Total survey	First priority	69%	11%	11%	3%	2%	3%
	Mean rank	1.68	3.12	3.30	4.03	4.39	4.45
Local authority nominees	First priority	65%	11%	14%	4%	2%	4%
	Mean rank	1.80	3.23	3.22	3.97	4.41	4.32
Voluntary organisation nominees	First priority	73%	11%	9%	3%	3%	2%
	Mean rank	1.56	2.99	3.39	4.05	4.37	4.58
RHA nominees	First priority	72%	13%	9%	2%	3%	1%
	Mean rank	1.57	3.13	3.27	4.15	4.34	4.50
Professional and Managerial	First priority	78%	9%	7%	3%	1%	2%
	Mean rank	1.43	3.05	3.37	4.01	4.49	4.59
White collar	First priority	63%	12%	13%	5%	3%	3%
	Mean rank	1.85	3.20	3.24	3.99	4.27	4.41
Blue collar	First priority	51%	18%	18%	3%	4%	6%
	Mean rank	2.08	3.17	3.24	4.08	4.27	4.15
Occupation in health, social and other public services	First priority	76%	11%	6%	3%	2%	2%
	Mean rank	1.50	2.97	3.45	3.97	4.53	4.52
'Other' occupation	First priority	64%	12%	15%	4%	3%	3%
	Mean rank	1.80	3.22	3.19	4.07	4.08	4.40

3.5   GENERAL ASSESSMENT OF HEALTH SERVICES

	Good %	Adequate %	Unsatis-factory %		Not stated
Total survey	32	50	18	100% (N = 3,050)	458 13% (N = 3,508)
	Very satisfied %	Quite satisfied %	Not very satisfied %	Not at all satisfied %	Don't know
NOP Survey[1]	30	51	15	4 100% (N = 1,677)	34 2% (N = 1,711)

1. N.O.P. Political Bulletin September 1974 p. 15.

3.6   DIFFERENCES IN THE GENERAL ASSESSMENT OF HEALTH SERVICES BY SOCIAL CHARACTERISTICS

	Good %	Adequate %	Unsatis-factory %		Not stated
Total sample	32	50	18	100% (N = 3,050)	458 13% (N = 3,508)
Professional and Managerial	30	53	16	100% (N = 1,638)	261 14% (N = 1,899)
White collar	34	48	18	100% (N = 825)	126 13% (N = 951)
Blue collar	33	46	21	100% (N = 475)	52 10% (N = 527)
Male	32	48	20	100% (N = 1,764)	243 12% (N = 2,007)
Female	32	53	15	100% (N = 1,277)	212 14% (N = 1,489)
Age under 35	13	50	38	100% (N = 268)	56 17% (N = 324)
35 – 54	27	53	20	100% (N = 1,459)	223 13% (N = 1,682)
55 and over	41	47	12	100% (N = 1,301)	175 12% (N = 1,476)

3.7 DIFFERENCES IN THE GENERAL ASSESSMENT OF HEALTH SERVICES BY ROLE AND EXPERIENCE

	Good %	Adequate %	Unsatis- factory %		Not stated
Total sample	32	50	18	100% (N = 3,050)	458 13% (N = 3,508)
1st priority of CHC role to:					
Channel	37	51	13	100% (N = 1,019)	133 11% (N = 1,152)
Represent	28	51	21	100% (N = 1,809)	251 12% (N = 2,060)
Understand	47	39	14	100% (N = 79)	11 12% (N = 90)
Occupation in health, social and other public services	29	52	19	100% (N = 1,241)	208 14% (N = 1,449)
Local authority nominees	32	50	19	100% (N = 1,433)	182 11% (N = 1,615)
Voluntary organisation nominees	31	51	17	100% (N = 1,126)	197 15% (N = 1,323)
RHA nominees	34	49	16	100% (N = 486)	78 14% (N = 564)
No previous health service experience	27	53	19	100% (N = 1,752)	330 16% (N = 2,082)
Some previous health service experience	38	46	16	100% (N = 1,278)	123 9% (N = 1,401)

3.8 REGIONAL VARIATIONS IN ASSESSMENTS AND RESOURCES

	Assessment "Good" %	Rank order of "good"*	Revenue expenditure £ per capita 1975/6[1]	Rank order of expenditure§
East Anglia	34	6	48.0	12
Mersey	32	7	56.7	5
Northern	38	2	51.0	7
North East Thames	24	14	67.0	1
North West Thames	27	11	65.5	2
North Western	27	11	51.8	6
Oxford	30	8	48.4	10
South East Thames	not available		(63.5)	
South West Thames	28	9	65.0	4
South Western	42	1	49.2	9
Trent	27	11	44.7	14
Wales	37	5	65.3	3
Wessex	38	2	48.4	10
West Midlands	28	9	47.3	13
Yorkshire	38	2	50.4	8
Total:	32			

* Rank 1 = highest percentage assessing service as good.
§ Rank 1 = highest expenditure per capita.
1. Figures for the English regions and for Wales are taken from Hansard, 4 February 1976 and 10 February 1976 respectively.

3.9 ASSESSMENTS AND RESOURCES IN 14 SINGLE-DISTRICT AREAS

CHC district	Provision of resources £ per capita, 1972/3[1]	Good	Assessment of services:— Adequate	Unsatis- factory	Can't say	
		%	%	%		
Sandwell	17.14	12	44	44	2	11% (N = 18)
Rotherham	17.43	25	44	31	2	11% (N = 18)
Wigan	18.62	0	75	25	3	16% (N = 19)
North Tyneside	19.00	29	71	0	4	22% (N = 18)
Trafford	19.26	12	41	47	2	10% (N = 19)
Bury	20.00	21	63	16	5	21% (N = 24)
Barnsley	21.08	45	36	18	2	15% (N = 13)
Bolton	21.54	12	75	12	2	11% (N = 18)
Hillingdon	22.51	47	60	0	5	25% (N = 20)
Doncaster	23.27	46	47	5	3	14% (N = 22)
Cornwall	25.10	35	65	0	—	(N = 20)
Gateshead	25.48	48	43	10	—	(N = 21)
Newcastle	29.91	33	67	0	6	25% (N = 24)
Salford	33.69	35	59	6	2	10% (N = 19)
National Total	£27.31	32	50	18	458	13% (N = 3,050)

1. Taken from J. H. Rickard 'Per capita expenditure of the English Area Health Authorities' *British Medical Journal* 31 January 1976. The national total for per capita spending is therefore for England only, while that for the assessments is for England and Wales.

3.10 THE ASSESSMENT OF PARTICULAR PROBLEMS IN THE HEALTH SERVICE

	Urgent problem %	Some problem %	No problem %		Can't say and not stated (N = 3,508)
Long-stay hospitals	39	54	7	100% (N = 2,634)	874 25%
Transport	29	61	10	100% (N = 2,547)	961 27%
Domiciliary services	23	69	8	100% (N = 2,431)	1,077 31%
General hospital services	22	66	12	100% (N = 2,806)	702 20%
Dental services	16	52	32	100% (N = 2,196)	1,312 37%
General practice	9	64	26	100% (N = 2,573)	935 27%
Pharmaceutical services	8	44	48	100% (N = 2,018)	1,490 42%

3.11 DIFFERENCES IN THE ASSESSMENT OF PARTICULAR HEALTH SERVICE PROBLEMS DISTRIBUTION OF 'URGENT PROBLEM'

	Long stay hospitals %	Transport %	Domi-ciliary services %	General hospital services %	Dental services %	General practice %	Pharma-ceutical services %
Total sample	39	29	23	22	16	9	8
Men	36	25	20	25	15	11	8
Women	43	34	27	22	19	8	8
Local authority nominees	36	28	21	22	16	11	10
Voluntary organisation nominees	42	31	27	21	17	8	6
RHA nominees	38	26	21	23	17	8	6
Age under 35	47	30	30	30	26	18	13
35 – 54	39	32	23	22	16	9	8
55 +	37	25	21	20	14	7	7
Professional and Managerial	39	30	24	20	17	9	6
White collar	38	28	25	22	15	9	8
Blue collar	38	25	18	24	17	11	11

Respondents who did not reply or could not say are excluded from these percentages. The figures show the proportion of positive respondents who assessed the particular service as an urgent problem.

3.12   REGIONAL DISTRIBUTION OF THE ASSESSMENT OF URGENT HEALTH SERVICE PROBLEMS

	Long stay hospitals %	Transport %	Domi-ciliary services %	General hospital services %	Dental services %	General practice %	Pharma-ceutical services %	Total for all services %
East Anglia	29	42	22	15	36	5	7	23
Mersey	35	27	17	24	8	10	5	19
Northern	31	24	20	16	7	4	4	16
North East Thames	45	33	33	26	27	15	12	28
North West Thames	48	34	33	17	33	13	5	27
North Western	40	21	30	21	16	14	8	22
Oxford	38	40	27	28	20	10	8	26
South East Thames				Not available				
South West Thames	35	39	22	17	13	8	1	20
South Western	39	20	18	22	7	4	11	18
Trent	45	28	24	28	11	13	15	24
Wales	37	31	17	17	15	7	6	19
Wessex	33	27	23	14	9	1	4	16
West Midlands	43	31	19	38	14	12	11	25
Yorkshire	34	16	22	11	16	8	9	17
Total:	39	29	23	22	16	9	8	

Respondents who did not reply or could not say are excluded from these percentages. The figures show the proportion of positive respondents who assessed the particular service as an urgent problem.

3.13   PRIORITIES FOR GROUPS

	Mean rank	Distribution of the first priority ranking* %
Mentally ill	3.68	16
Elderly	3.80	20
Mentally handicapped	3.91	16
Acutely ill patients	4.04	22
Physically handicapped	4.28	6
Children	4.73	6
Ordinary patients	5.22	12
Maternity	6.17	2

* Respondents who did not reply are excluded from these figures. The percentages show the proportion of positive respondents who gave the particular group a first priority rating.

The first priority was ranked (1)

3.14 DIFFERENCES IN THE PRIORITIES GIVEN TO PARTICULAR GROUPS BY CLASS AND NOMINATING GROUPS

		Mentally ill	Elderly	Mentally handicapped	Acutely ill patients	Physically handicapped	Children	Ordinary patients	Maternity
Total Survey	First priority	16%	20%	16%	22%	6%	6%	12%	2%
	Mean rank	3.68	3.80	3.91	4.04	4.28	4.73	5.22	6.17
Local authority nominees	First priority	16%	20%	15%	24%	6%	8%	11%	2%
	Mean rank	3.77	3.96	3.95	3.87	4.23	4.61	5.37	6.07
Voluntary organisation nominees	First priority	16%	21%	17%	20%	8%	6%	11%	1%
	Mean rank	3.55	3.73	3.85	4.26	4.24	4.81	5.19	6.27
RHA nominees	First priority	15%	26%	14%	24%	4%	4%	14%	1%
	Mean rank	3.76	3.50	3.96	4.02	4.52	4.93	4.85	6.24
Professional and managerial	First priority	17%	22%	16%	20%	5%	6%	13%	1%
	Mean rank	3.60	3.64	3.88	4.34	4.36	4.81	4.97	6.25
White collar	First priority	16%	18%	14%	26%	8%	7%	11%	1%
	Mean rank	3.72	4.05	4.00	3.70	4.20	4.64	5.39	6.14
Blue collar	First priority	12%	18%	18%	25%	8%	7%	10%	2%
	Mean rank	3.97	3.91	3.91	3.57	4.15	4.62	5.70	6.02
Occupation in health, social and other public services	First priority	17%	23%	15%	20%	6%	5%	12%	1%
	Mean rank	3.54	3.63	3.85	4.32	4.30	4.88	5.04	6.30

3.15 DIFFERENCES IN THE PRIORITIES GIVEN TO PARTICULAR GROUPS BY VOLUNTARY ORGANISATION MEMBERS

		Mentally ill	Elderly	Mentally handicapped	Acutely ill patients	Physically handicapped	Children	Ordinary patients	Maternity
Total Survey	First priority	16%	20%	16%	22%	6%	6%	12%	2%
	Mean rank	3.68	3.80	3.91	4.04	4.28	4.73	5.22	6.17
Members of organisations concerned with: —									
Mentally handicapped	First priority	15%	15%	33%	17%	4%	6%	9%	2%
	Mean rank	3.47	3.88	3.10	4.20	4.43	4.86	5.64	6.28
Mental health	First priority	31%	18%	19%	13%	4%	5%	7%	2%
	Mean rank	2.85	3.66	3.38	4.74	4.42	5.10	5.41	6.33
Physically handicapped	First priority	11%	17%	16%	23%	14%	5%	12%	1%
	Mean rank	3.89	4.02	3.94	3.95	3.71	4.77	5.36	6.24
The elderly	First priority	11%	23%	14%	24%	8%	7%	12%	2%
	Mean rank	3.94	3.53	3.99	3.83	4.19	4.80	5.35	6.27
Children and maternity	First priority	16%	19%	18%	20%	4%	8%	12%	2%
	Mean rank	3.56	3.81	3.73	4.33	4.34	4.58	5.21	6.23

113

4

Aspirations, activities and frustrations

So far the CHC members have been analysed in terms of who they are and what they think. In this chapter we look at representation as an activity: at what the CHC members actually did in their first year in office. In doing so, we look at three related sets of questions. First, how do they define in practice their role as consumer representatives — a role which is capable of many interpretations[1]. To what extent do they act as spokesmen for the consumer, eliciting and amplifying the views of the public and of the patient? And how far do they act more broadly as the trustees of the consumer interest, making judgments on behalf of the population at large? Second, what does the first-year experience of the CHCs indicate about the structure of the reorganised NHS? Does the fact that CHCs are outside the managerial hierarchy mean that they have a different approach to the problems of the NHS to that of administrators and members of health authorities? And how far does this role impose frictional costs on the administration and create a sense of frustration among CHC members? Third, what do the activities of the CHCs show about the shortcomings of the NHS? To what extent does the existence of a body of consumer representatives — however they may define their role — provide new insights about the provision of services?

These questions are easier to ask than to answer. There are the problems of research method. Given the heterogeneity of the CHCs, in respect of both their own characteristics and of their environments, the traditional case study approach is only of limited help. It may deepen the understanding of specific local circumstances, but does not permit generalisation about the institution as a whole. Equally, as noted in the introduction, CHCs have so far only had a very short life, and it would be misleading to draw large conclusions from the struggle of a new institution seeking to establish itself in a health service caught in the turmoil of reorganisation.

This chapter is, therefore, analytical but not statistical. It uses as its raw material the annual reports which the CHCs are obliged to publish: just over half the CHCs in England and Wales made these reports available to us. In addition, the discussion is informed by closer contacts with a number of individual CHCs[2]. But since annual reports must be read with a certain scepticism — they are, after all, exercises in public relations and may reflect the personality of the chairman or secretary as much as the activities of the CHC — no attempt is made to translate their contents into any kind of numerical assessment about how many of them are doing what. The intention, instead, is to use them to delineate the kinds of problems and to define the types of behaviour that were illustrated by the activities of CHCs in their first year. This approach has the additional advantage of drawing attention to some of the general issues which are relevant to consumer representation in all public services. These issues, in turn, illuminate the policy options for the future which are the subject of the next and final chapter.

A one-side love affair

The annual reports of CHCs come in all shapes and sizes. Some are glossy, printed pamphlets which would not be out of place in a trade-exhibition. Others are home-made affairs, typed, duplicated and stapled in the CHC office. Some are introduced in stately prose by their chairmen, seizing on this opportunity to broadcast their views on the state of the world and of the NHS. Others are quietly business-like. Some are barely more than a record of meetings held, apologies received and business done; others contain detailed descriptions of visits made to hospitals, complaints received, resources available and discussions held. Just to look through them is to become convinced of the diversity among CHCs.

Yet despite this diversity, one theme runs through the reports: a lament about the frustrating, disappointingly one-sided love affair which CHCs have had with the public. Almost two-thirds of CHC members, as noted in the previous chapter, see it as their role to represent the community. Inevitably, therefore, one of the first tasks which CHCs set themselves was to make their existence known: for how can you represent that mysterious entity, the community, if none of its members even know of your existence? Posters were put on display in Post Offices and other public places; leaflets were distributed; advertisements were put in the local press; the public were invited to attend CHC meetings; councillors and secretaries addressed Women's Institutes and Pensioners' Clubs. But though the extent and the enthusiasm of the campaign may have varied, the result seems to have been the same almost everywhere: the public obstinately refused to take much notice. A number of small surveys — conducted somewhat prematurely perhaps — showed overwhelming ignorance of the existence of CHCs[3]; and many of the CHC reports are eloquent of disappointment:

"In spite of the publicity efforts, the majority of the public and many within the health service have still not heard of the Community Health Council. The public have been encouraged to come forward with their ideas, suggestions, comments, but the response so far has been disappointing. No members of the public have attended a meeting..." (North Derbyshire)

"Meetings of the Council have been held at different venues... in order to publicise the existence of the Council throughout the district and to encourage the public to attend meetings in their immediate area. This has not met with a large measure of success" (East Surrey)

"It is deplorable that the creation of a consumer body in any area of such public concern has not been extensively advertised nationally... we feel that our budget allocation of £2,651 for publicity, postage, stationery, equipment, maintenance, cleaning, members' travelling expenses, etc., is a severe limitation on our scope to inform the public that we exist to serve them" (South Hammersmith)

"The meetings of the Community Health Council are open to the public, but as yet not many have availed themselves of the opportunity to attend" (Great Yarmouth)

"Most people in the district will not even have heard of the Community Health Council and it is clear that the Council must now start to establish its identity within the community" (Eastern Liverpool)

The litany of complaints about inadequate public knowledge and response could be greatly extended. But the picture conveyed — of CHCs ignored by the communities which they are supposed to represent — is exaggerated. A few CHCs do have a success story to tell. In certain circumstances, people do take notice of their existence: when the CHC offers a platform for community and group grievances and when it associates itself with a locally salient issue.

Some CHCs have managed to make themselves the focus of public attention by organising campaigns:

> "A large task during the year has been the organisation of a petition to the Secretary of State. This was deemed the correct role of the Council as community representative when rebuilding of the General Infirmary, Leeds, was threatened. The work was hard but the results proved encouraging. The Yorkshire Evening Post supported the petition and their unstinting and magnificent coverage was most sincerely appreciated. Although at the time of this report there is no official answer, the project brought to the notice of the public the work of the Council. This has served to explain to the public our role in the Health Service and illustrated to all who work in the Service that we have an important part to play in its development" (Western Leeds)

More usually, and less spectacularly, CHCs — sometimes prompted by the Parish Council — have arranged meetings to discuss specific local issues. For instance, Swindon CHC organised a public meeting to discuss whether there should be a pharmacy within a new Health Centre or whether "the public would be better served by a chemist's shop which it was proposed to open in an adjacent shopping arcade". In another case, the CHC reacted to local concern about a Health Centre:

> "In April 1975 a new health centre opened in Fountayne Road. Some time later the local ward Labour Party approached us with the idea of holding a public meeting to tell people what goes on in a health centre. There was a mixed reaction from the health professionals to this idea. Over 2,000 leaflets were distributed and the local paper carried a small item. Fifty people attended. Much of the discussion centred on the administration of the centre which had gone through a difficult time..." (City and Hackney)

All this would seem to indicate that CHCs attract attention to the extent that they provide a specific service to the public: when members of the community feel that they, as individuals, will get something in return for their investment of time or interest. The problem, in other words, is not to create a blanket public awareness of the existence of CHCs: this is to assume — wrongly — that people will go on taking an interest out of a general sense of civic duty. It is to make sure that people will be able to find out about their existence if, and when, they have need of some specific service provided by the CHC.

This, in any case, is true of all public bodies. When, some years ago, a study revealed that hardly anyone had heard of the consumer consultative committees attached to the nationalised industries, there was widespread dismay and consternation[4]. In fact, ignorance about public services and public bodies is the norm. For example, when a survey carried out for the Commission on the Constitution[5] asked people to name those responsible for running primary schools, the hospital service, the electricity board and the postal services, only 28% of those interviewed got three or more of the answers right. Over a third gave only one or no correct reply. Similarly, when the Maud Committee on the Management of Local Government asked local authorities how many members of the public attended council meetings[6], 109 out of 151 replied none (excluding school children and other organised parties). What matters in these circumstances, surely, is that people should be able to use the telephone and the telephone directory — not that they should constantly be using the instrument or memorising all the numbers. It is the ability to use the network, when the occasion demands it, which is crucial — not a continued, routine interest in its operations, irrespective of specific needs and concerns. In the case of the NHS most of the people are satisfied most of the time, as we have seen and there is no reason to expect them to invest time and trouble in paying attention to the activities of CHCs on a routine basis[7]. They are, in a sense, more rational in their lack of interest than CHC members are in their belief that the public ought to be interested.

This may be an uncomfortable conclusion for CHC members. If they cannot speak for the community — in the sense of conveying the views of the population concerned — from where do they draw their authority? Why, in that case, should anyone listen to them? In contrast to elected councillors — who may well claim to carry authority by the mere fact of having been voted into office, even if subsequently they remain totally isolated from the public — CHC members have to create their own links with the community. How is it possible to conceive of CHCs injecting an element of democracy into the NHS — whatever may be meant by that — if the *demos,* when it comes to the point, obstinately ignore the existence of this new institution?

At the extremes, there are two strategies for coping with this dilemma — both, in practice, characteristic of only a very few CHCs but worth examining all the same since they illustrate the range of behaviour. The first is to adopt the trustee position: to view the CHC as representing, in the words of the South East Cumbria annual report, the "informed and considered opinion" of the community. "The Council remembers", the report continues, "that its duty to protect and foster local health interests may not always mean 'taking the popular line'." But even this CHC spent a considerable amount of energy on publicising its existence. Alternatively, at the other extreme, there is the populist position: in this view even the members of the CHCs are tainted apologists for the *status quo* unless they are in direct communion with "ordinary people". To quote the chairman's introduction to one report:

> "It is a matter of regret that the mass of working people and their families who use the health services have still not heard of CHCs. Until such people can come forward to speak for that large majority, those of us who occupy these seats can only do so undemocratically. CHCs cannot therefore 'democratise' anything let alone the vast hierarchical NHS."
> (Wandsworth and East Merton)

The same report provides insight into the problems that can arise in a CHC where members are militantly self-conscious about their role and bring into the open some of the tensions and ambiguities implicit in the system:

> "During the first few months some members wondered aloud why they had been 'chosen'. Others did not doubt their own right to membership but appeared to question the legitimacy of others and these attitudes seem to have persisted. Members are expected to represent the consumer in the Health Service but there is as yet little agreement amongst ourselves exactly how this may be achieved. There is competitiveness regarding who really represents whom and how many of them. Local Borough Councillors, both Conservative and Labour, argue that they are the most representative as they speak for the electorate. Grass-roots community workers argue that they see more local people and their families than anybody else. Others present themselves as 'individual consumers' and feel that they are representative of average patients. Although all three of these strands of information and experience are useful the effect of mixing them together is quite often disastrous...Thus the monthly meetings have often been unpleasant affairs with angry verbal clashes".

Most CHCs are not racked so self-consciously by doubts as to why they were created, or about their legitimacy, nor are they waiting for the people to take over the council chamber. Instead, many CHCs have been exploring other ways of searching out information about local opinion and local needs.

One such way is to conduct public opinion surveys. And this is what a number of CHCs have done with varying degrees of sophistication. Some have done so to test whether vociferously expressed opinions represent the silent majority:

> "...the Chairman of the CHC arranged with the Wellington County Secondary School for Girls in Timperley for the fifth and sixth year students to undertake a survey to determine the views of Timperley residents about the Health Centre. Using a prepared questionnaire the students interviewed 599 members of the public in different parts of Timperley... An analysis of these questionnaires indicated that of the 599 people interviewed only some 20% regarded the Centre as a 'waste of money' while 79.97% regarded it as either 'useful' or 'essential'. On the basis of this evidence it appeared that the opposition to this scheme which had been noted prior to the survey, particularly as expressed in letters in the local papers, had been the views of a vocal minority. The proposal to build the Timperley Health Centre was approved and supported by the CHC". (Trafford)

Others have done so to find out the priorities of local consumers. For example, East Dorset CHC distributed questionnaires at meetings which asked: "If you had control over local health services, but only had sufficient money to spend on maintaining or developing ten of the following 25 services, which ten would you choose?" Interestingly, the first 264 people so questioned gave the accident and emergency services as their first priority, followed by the GP services, with the geriatric services and domiciliary nursing care in third place. The mentally ill and handicapped do not find any place in the first seven priorities. It would be wrong to draw any large conclusions from a small survey in one district, but the example does indicate a potential dilemma for CHCs. How are they to react if their own personal priorities — which, as shown in the previous chapter, tend to reflect elite attitudes and support governmental policies for giving first claim to the most disadvantaged groups in the population — come into conflict with the priorities of the populations whom they represent? How are they to act if (as seems possible) the local population is primarily concerned to improve the availability of acute services? Do they, then, insist that they have access to information and insights denied to the community as a whole or do they simply echo the majority view? The dilemma is, of course, common to all representatives; but it is particularly acute for CHC members because it is not even clear in what respects 'they are meant to be representative.

So far most CHC members have been behaving as though it is up to them to generate their own information and make their own judgments, rather than relying on the input from the public at large. In this respect, they emphatically and overwhelmingly do not see themselves as spokesmen of the community but as guardians of the community's interests, and as such responsible for investigating and inspecting the provision of health care in the district. Nearly all CHCs have set up teams of members to visit the local health care facilities, though there are considerable variations in the enthusiasm shown for this activity and in the detailed arrangements made. Some CHCs have teams for particular geographical areas; others have teams assigned to specific health care sectors; many have teams for the different health care groups, like the elderly or the mentally ill. In short, they are representing the ordinary citizen not in the sense of echoing his views but of doing what he would be doing, given the time and the opportunity to inquire into, and form a judgment about, the state of the local health services. This further helps to explain, and justify, the anxiety of CHCs to establish more links with the public. If they see themselves as having an educative function — if one of their roles is to be a sort of proxy inspector of health services on behalf of the consumer, reporting back on problems and issues — then it is clearly essential to be in touch with the audience which is being educated.

One way of keeping in touch is, as argued previously, to "plug" into the existing communications network of the community. And, as demonstrated in Chapter 2, CHC members do bring with them a fund of experience in a variety of roles, whether in voluntary organisations or in local government. But these links, in turn, create new problems, to judge from the first year's record of the CHCs. The price of recruiting strategic public persons — i.e. CHC members who are part of a variety of networks — may be that these are the familiar, over-busy committee man or woman, unable to give up much time to the work of Community Health Councils. The following quotation sums up a frequent theme:

> "The local authority members with committee experience, their knowledge of local government business, and in regular contact with their constituents, have proved invaluable to the work of the Council. However, membership of a Community Health Council has involved far more than any of the members envisaged when they were first appointed

— so much so that four District Councillors who were heavily committed to local government work have found it necessary to resign from the CHC". (South Nottingham)

In Oxfordshire, ten out of the 30 CHC members resigned in the first year: eight out of the ten being local authority nominees. And even where local authority nominees did not resign on such a massive scale, there is widespread evidence that they were not able to participate in the work of CHCs as frequently as other members. Scunthorpe CHC, for example, reported that the average attendance record for local authority nominees was only 48%, as against 67% and 70% for voluntary organisation and RHA nominees respectively. Similarly, Huddersfield CHC pointed out that the attendance figures for local authority members were 57%, as against 82% and 77% for the other two groups.

The problem of attendance and of a high wastage rate may well turn out to be a passing phenomenon. It may reflect the fact that, in the first instance, many of the local authority members were press-ganged into taking on this additional chore, at a time when no one could be sure how much work would be involved. Given more knowledge about the job itself, and given an increasing self-selection by people who are actually interested in the health service, these difficulties may solve themselves. In any event, it is impossible to know — in the absence of comparative information — whether the problems of the CHCs in this respect are in any way different from those of other bodies dependent on voluntary, unpaid participation: while local authorities at least offer attendance allowances to their members, CHCs can only offer expenses and loss of earnings payments.

But it is also possible that some of the difficulties of CHCs — in retaining their members and persuading them to take a full part in their work — spring from the way in which the councils have defined their function. To the extent that the CHCs see it as their role to generate more information — to inquire for themselves, instead of merely acting as part of an on-going communications network — so they impose greater burdens on their members. As their spokesman role merges into a wider investigatory role, so they will inevitably demand more commitment from their members. This, in turn, would suggest that these members may increasingly have to be recruited on the basis of their readiness to give up time rather than because they are, in some sense or other, representative of the population. If the functions of the CHCs expand, so the number of men and women available to sit on them may shrink.

Consuming interest v. organisation interest

One of the implicit assumptions behind the creation of CHCs was that the interests of the consumer of medical care are different from those of the providers and organisers of health services. In turn, this suggests that the interests of patient and public have, somehow, got to be protected against doctors, administrators and the other professionals within the NHS. But this is not, of course, how the health service professionals perceive the situation. They cannot do so without abandoning their view of themselves: for what distinguishes a professional from a shop-keeper is precisely the fact that his duty lies in doing for the client what professional knowledge and professional ethics dictate, not what the client wants[8]. To a degree, the ideologies of consumerism and of professionalism are inevitably in conflict. And one of the ways in which to explore the first-year activities of the CHC is to look upon these as an attempt to explore and define the neutral zone between consumerism and professionalism, where it is possible to voice the interests of health service users without overtly challenging those of the health service providers.

In the outcome, there were few open clashes between CHCs and the professions. Still, there was enough evidence of professional sensitivity to suggest that this absence of conflict may have owed more to the care with which most CHCs proceeded than to a readiness among the professions to welcome the activities of this new institution. For example, an inquiry by one CHC about the work of an obstetric department, and in particular about the medical criteria for deciding about the induction of labour, provoked a sharp reaction from the Joint Consultants Committee, which represents all hospital consultants[9]. The Committee totally rejected the implied suggestion that a CHC might be entitled to ask for information from a doctor. The consultants asked the Chief Medical Officer of the DHSS to give CHCs firm guidance: "It must be made clear that the CHC as such has no power to compel any professional member of NHS staff to appear before it, or to provide it with information. Furthermore, the provision of any information by an area health authority to the CHC which could lead to debate therein about matters of clinical judgment of consultant or other staff was not a duty of the AHA, and that discussion in a CHC of the performance or practice of consultants in the district was not within a council's terms of reference".

Nor were the consultants alone in taking this view. The Confederation of Health Service Employees, which includes nurses and other staff, and the medical profession usually appear together in the headlines only when they are at loggerheads with each other. But they were at one when it came to CHCs. Mr Albert Spanswick, COHSE's Secretary-General, was emphatic about the need to fence in the activities of CHCs [10]: "Community Health Councils were established in the reorganised service to play a useful part in monitoring the needs of the community to the Authority. Their members must not, however, be allowed to visit hospitals, health centres, homes and so on, to enquire into the work of staff or into professional procedures; in my view, such licence would only result in a deterioration of industrial relations, bringing with it loss of confidence in the whole structure. Firm guidelines are therefore, in my view, essential to facilitate good relations between staff, patients and the CHC".

But it is not only doctors and nurses who look upon themselves as professionals, and as such resent anything which could be construed as a lay invasion of their territory or as a challenge to their expertise. Administrators, too, perceive themselves as professionals. And there is some evidence that they believe at least part of their professionalism to lie precisely in their ability to define and represent the public or community interest: they may therefore come to see community representatives as filling the role which they themselves are already playing [11]. This is one reason why it has been argued that it is just as important to have a "representative bureaucracy" — in the sense of mirroring the values and social composition of the population — as to have representative elected bodies [12].

Additionally, administrators can reasonably claim to know more about consumer wants and grievances than representative bodies like CHCs. This is less paradoxical than it sounds. Most people, if they have any problems or grievances will, in the first place, approach those responsible for the particular service involved. This can be seen from the results of a survey on community attitudes carried out in 1968 on behalf of the Royal Commission on Local Government [13]. The survey showed a sample of electors a list of public services and asked them: "Suppose you wanted to make an enquiry or complaint about any of these services, or any others, who would you get in touch with first of all?". Over two-thirds of those interviewed said that they would approach an official, while a mere 17% mentioned an elected representative of one kind or another. Only if the first contact fails to bring satisfaction are service consumers likely to contact a representative rather than an administrator. This would suggest that, to the extent that CHCs view themselves as purveyors of information about consumer opinion, they may be perceived as rivals by the administrators.

Given these considerations, it is not surprising that a survey of NHS administrators carried out in 1975 showed considerable scepticism about CHCs [14]. Distance lent indulgence to the views of regional administrators: three-quarters of these thought that CHCs were likely to be effective as consumer councils. But propinquity brought disenchantment: of the district administrators, i.e. those most likely to be in direct touch with CHCs, only 29% took this favourable view, while over 40% postponed judgment. Among the criticisms made of CHCs was that these tended to see themselves as part of management, that they exerted power without responsibility, that there was a tendency for them to be used as political platforms, and that it was doubtful how representative they were.

The stage would, therefore, appear to be set for a confrontation between those working in the NHS and the CHCs. But yet a further set of characters is involved: the members of Area Health Authorities — originally appointed, it will be remembered, to carry out an exclusively managerial role which became somewhat more representative when the 1974 Labour Government changed the composition of the AHAs. Here, too, there is some evidence of an overlap — threatening friction — in the functions of the AHA members, as perceived by themselves, and those of the CHC members. A survey of both AHA and CHC members, carried out in one Area [15] found that both "gave virtually identical replies to a question about how they saw their main job (both groups asserting that their main job was to 'guide developments in the area' *and* 'to safeguard the interests of the patient')". And although this survey was small in scale, the results are consistent with what might have been expected from the modifications made to the original model of the reorganised NHS which — as noted in the first chapter — resulted in blurring the functions of the AHAs and the CHCs.

In the event, the predictable conflict between NHS managers and CHCs did take place, although it was not as universal or bitter as the above, schematic analysis might suggest. The two main causes for friction are summed up in the following quotation:

> "Like any new body, the Community Health Council has been trying to discover what services are available... Some difficulty has been found in obtaining this sort of information from the Area Health Authority, particularly about community services, and this lack of information has hindered the Council's work. In addition to general information, the Council have found it difficult to obtain specific information relevant to plans for providing health centres and were informed by the Area

Management Team that information about current services provided in particular areas was not readily available and that, in any case, information about catchment areas to health centres was not really relevant for the Council's purposes...

The Area Health Authority are obliged to consult the Community Health Council when considering any plans for extension, change of use or closure of health service premises. Most of the consultation to date has been at a very late stage, often after requests from the CHC, and at a stage where the comments of the Community Health Council cannot be incorporated into the plans". (Sunderland)

The Sunderland Area Health Authority, in turn, replied to the CHC's comments with some asperity:

"...it was anticipated that the Community Health Council would recognise that, as advised in HRC(74)4 paragraph 31, the first duty of National Health Service staff was to meet the needs of patients and in the period following reorganisation the Authority would be incompletely staffed and under heavy pressure. The Area Health Authority accepted the need for a close working relationship with the Community Health Council in order to achieve the aims of the Council but it soon became apparent that the methods of achieving them led to differing interpretations of the advice as between the CHC and the Authority. This would not have mattered greatly had it not been for the reaction of the Community Health Council in these circumstances taking an extreme line and quickly dissipating the atmosphere of goodwill which had existed in the initial stages. The situation was highlighted by the use of the Press to gain headlines and the public criticism of many aspects of the service without having undertaken a careful investigation...

...the reason for the critical attitude by the Council towards consultation results from the difference in view as to what is meant by this term. The Authority has the impression from the terms of the correspondence that the Community Health Council wishes to be involved in the actual membership of the various committees set up for managerial purposes e.g. the Health Care Planning Teams. The Council also seem to see it as their role to make detailed comments on day-to-day management questions within hospitals and clinics following their visits, and also on sketch plans submitted to them for general comment: the Area Authority does not see this as within the role of the Community Health Council".

This exchange has been quoted at length because it illustrates most of the problems involved in the relationship between CHCs and health authorities. In this particular instance, the arena of conflict was a single district AHA; in the majority of cases the CHCs were dealing primarily with the District Management Team in multi-district areas, with the AHA in the background rather than in the forefront of the argument. But the themes were much the same everywhere: lack of information and failure to consult. The complaints about lack of information take many forms. Some CHCs protested against being denied the minutes of the DMT (which, unlike the AHA, meets in private and has no statutory obligation to publish an account of its proceedings). Others grumbled about the inadequacy of statistics about the use of local services. Again, as some CHCs were quick to point out, the word "consult" is capable of many interpretations. It can mean anything from going through the formal motions of seeking the views of CHCs about decisions that have already been taken to involving them in the deliberative processes leading up to the final decisions: and while some health authorities clearly took the former view, all CHCs argued for the latter interpretation :

> "Whilst the Council appreciate the natural caution of professional officers in admitting amateurs to their councils, they must ask that time is given to the Council for proper consideration of plans which are put before them — participating in the formulation of plans might in the long run prove to be the only expeditious way of achieving this. If we are to make a meaningful contribution to planning, we need to be brought into the planning process at as early a stage as possible". (Burnley, Pendle and Rossendale)

To a degree, such conflicts are rooted in the ambiguities of the relationship between CHCs and the NHS organisational system. CHCs may have a right to information, but how far do they have a right to demand that there should be an extra investment of effort to obtain statistics which are not available off-the-peg? From the point of view of those within the NHS organisational system, demands for such statistics may well be seen as the imposition of extra burdens by people who do not have to live with the consequences of the additional work they have generated. From the point of view of CHC members, a reluctance to carry out special surveys or dig out figures may well be perceived as the defensive reaction of administrators who believe that knowledge is power. Again, the demand to take part in the decision-process — rather than being asked to comment on the final outcome of it — may seem, to the managers of the NHS, like an attempt to usurp their function.

Even so, it is possible that the first year reports of the CHCs give an exaggerated impression of friction. This was a period in which both the CHCs and the NHS authorities were learning their job in a newly organised service. Additionally, there were a number of practical difficulties. Many AHAs and DMTs were themselves short of the staff needed to collect information: so trying to satisfy the curiosity of CHCs may well have been resented with special force in these circumstances. Similarly, the process of consultation was complicated by the fact that the new health authorities were themselves for the most part simply implementing decisions which they had inherited: CHCs were, in effect, trying to climb onto a moving train rolling along predestined lines — as most of them recognised by accepting, albeit reluctantly, the various plans and proposals put in front of them. Additionally, and most frustratingly for both the CHCs and all health authorities, the introduction of the "planning system" was repeatedly postponed by the DHSS. The planning system was the name given — in the Grey Book and elsewhere (16) — to the formal framework for taking decisions about the allocation of resources at all levels of the NHS and the process by which the various administrative tiers were to engage in a dialogue about their objectives and priorities. As such, it was supposed to be the cornerstone of the reorganised NHS. But during the period under consideration, it remained on the designer's test bench. Instead of being involved in a new type of long-term planning as promised, CHC members — like everyone else — found themselves engaged in the depressingly familiar business of discussing day-to-day tactical decisions without any idea about what the day after tomorrow would bring. Too many people found themselves, in effect, involved in planning too little: fighting over a non-existent bone.

Not all CHCs were equally anxious to take part in the planning processes, such as they were. The differences in attitude come out most clearly in the views taken by various CHCs about their relationship with the Health Care Planning Teams. These Health Care Planning Teams — which were gradually being set up in the districts during the first year of the CHCs — are charged with identifying gaps in provision and opportunities for improvement in services for specific groups in the population, like the elderly, children, the mentally ill and handicapped. They are multi-disciplinary, and may include representatives of local authority services as well as a whole range of NHS staff. Given this wide membership, and given also that the groups covered by the Health Care Planning Teams were much the same as those where the CHC's voluntary organisation members had a special interest, it is not surprising that many councils sought to participate in their work. In some cases they knocked at an open door: they were invited either as full members or as observers. But in other cases, the door remained shut:

> "Sadly it would seem that we are not, at least in the present circumstances, going to have a permanent place on the Health Care Planning Teams. This really does seem to be a short-sighted decision... Indeed it would seem that the Health Care Planning Teams are to comprise solely Senior Officers. Surely, if Health Care Planning Teams are to plan sensibly and logically, they must have permanent members who are continually involved with the care of the patient on a daily basis. It is interesting to learn that a specially funded experimental Health Care Planning Team for the mentally handicapped found that all the information they had taken months to gather could have been obtained from talking to just one parent of a mentally handicapped child. The CHC make a plea to the DMT to remember that planning is not for Senior Staff alone, but must involve closely the people who are actually providing the Service, and also the consumer who receives that planned Service". (Mansfield and Newark)

Other CHCs took a more sceptical view, and some clearly felt that membership of such teams might compromise their independence:

> "In Bolton there is a feeling that membership of planning teams could dull the Council's critical edge. Nevertheless it is considered essential for the Community Health Council to know about plans in embryo, through regular meetings with planning teams..." (Bolton)

> "In 1975 for the first time CHC members have been invited to become contributing members of HCPTs: they have accepted this with mixed feelings, and have regarded the opportunity as an experiment for the first year. There are obvious dangers and difficulties of confidentiality, identification with management and lack of professional knowledge... Each member who attends HCPT meetings is backed by a 'mirror group' of three other CHC members with similar service interests, who can ensure that a properly representative view is being put over to HCPTs, and can identify areas of study where the CHC might be able to do some detailed work with the public". (West Dorset)

The DHSS took a recessive role in providing guidance about the relationship between CHCs and management. Little attempt was made to translate the general right of CHCs to information into specific guidelines about their entitlement to see particular documents. So it is not surprising, in an extreme case, to find the following comment:

"The lack of information given to the Council has been one of the most disappointing features of the year. Many members had naturally expected there would be an automatic feed-out of quite a lot of information to them. Unfortunately this has not happened. After a while government circulars did start to arrive but the only other regular source of written information were Area Health Authority Minutes with some supporting papers and Regional Health Authority Minutes with no supporting papers. There have been no Family Practitioner or District Management Team minutes received. There is no District Bulletin and there has been only one meeting between some members of the CHC and the District Management Team during the year. This means it is not possible to really know what is going on". (Darlington)

This example is of particular interest because Darlington Memorial Hospital was, subsequently, the subject of a special inquiry into four deaths at the psychiatric unit there. This report [17] was critical both of the District Administrator and, in a passing comment, of the local CHC: "We were surprised to find no evidence of visits to the unit by members of the Community Health Council and, it appears, that little or no information is passing between them in either direction". The Darlington inquiry also prompts the question of how much access CHCs should be given to the reports of the Hospital Advisory Service (now re-labelled Health Advisory Service) — an inspectorate in all but name, which reports directly to the Secretary of State [18]. The Darlington psychiatric unit, the report points out, had been visited in 1974 by a HAS team which had noted some of the weaknesses in its administrative arrangements. But "few of their recommendations appear to have been implemented, and in general their advice appears to have been ignored". This echoes the conclusions of a committee of inquiry into conditions at another hospital — St. Augustine's, near Canterbury, where yet again the report stressed the disregard of recommendations made by a HAS team [19] — and gives added point to the following complaint:

"The CHC has enquired as to the availability of the report of the Hospital Advisory Service team which has visited Guy's and St. Olave's Psychiatric Units, in order to ascertain what recommendations were made and what follow-up action has been taken. All efforts to procure this information have failed on the grounds that staff receive assurances about the confidential nature of HAS reports. If deficiencies were

> revealed, the Council is of the view that it would be in the best interests of the NHS and its management if the findings are made available. It can only invite suspicion of inadequacy to draw so close a veil of secrecy". (Guy's)

In this instance, the DHSS has provided some guidance to health authorities: Area Health Authorities *may* (our italics) "inform CHCs of the recommendations ... that the HAS has tendered in its reports" [20]. But leaving the decision to the discretion of the health authorities does not dispose of the underlying difficulty. If the role of CHCs is perceived to be to voice the views of the community — and just that — then clearly they have no need for any information except that which stems from patients and public. If, in contrast, CHCs are assigned a role in the planning process and in the assessment of services, then inevitably they will seek to arm themselves with specialist knowledge and to emancipate themselves from being entirely dependent on information supplied by those whose performance they may have to criticise. In these circumstances, giving health authorities permission to show a summary of the HAS recommendations to Community Health Councils — instead of making this mandatory — may not be a satisfactory solution.

It would be a mistake to conclude from these examples of friction that the introduction of CHCs has given institutional expression to the on-going conflict between the consumer interest and the producer interest in the NHS. The situation, as the experience of CHCs so far indicates, is more complex than this neat and familiar antithesis would suggest. First, in many instances producer and consumer interests are identical. Second, both producers and consumers are a very mixed bag; and there are competing and conflicting interests within each group. Instead of looking at their relationship in terms of a Cowboys and Indians conflict, it is therefore much more accurate to picture it as an elaborately choreographed ballet — with the dancers constantly changing partners and adopting new formations as the setting of the drama changes. The following quotations illustrate both points in turn:

> "The Council has given full support to the District Management Team's recommendation for a new District General Hospital and has been instrumental in having resolutions passed regarding this urgency by both the Reigate and Banstead Borough Council and the Tandridge District Council. Letters have also been sent from the Council to the three Members of Parliament... and the Council have sponsored a petition asking for support from hospital staff. At the same time the Council is

supporting a petition for a new District General Hospital sponsored by The Surrey Mirror, the Caterham Times and the Horley Adviser". (East Surrey)

"We were approached by the Consultant Dermatologist based at the Derbyshire Royal Infirmary about the services in the Derby area. He expressed his concern about the deterioration of these services and asked for our support in his efforts to secure improvements. It was understood that the appointment of an additional consultant had been approved, but that the necessary funds for this post had not been made available by the Regional Authority. As a result of our approach to the Area Authority, the Administrator sent a further reminder to the Regional Medical Officer drawing attention to the particular problems highlighted by the Consultant". (Central Derbyshire)

The first quotation underlines the fact that Community Health Councils and NHS staff have a shared interest, in any specific locality, to seek extra resources for their particular services — and, conversely, to resist any attempts to cut these back. CHCs provide the health service professionals with an opportunity to politicise the issue: to identify their own self-interest with that of the community as a whole. In these circumstances, the CHC may become significant as part of the political network: mobilising, as the example quoted shows, local authorities, local press and local MPs. This is not to suggest that there were no local constituencies for the health services before the CHCs were invented. But it emphasises their importance in offering a permanent platform for this constituency, and providing it with institutional visibility and an organisational framework.

The second quotation shows that the help of CHCs can also be invoked by individuals or interest groups within the NHS who are seeking support in the competition to attract extra resources. In other words, the CHCs do not face a monolithic NHS. They are themselves actors in a shifting world of coalitions, where there are a great many groups seeking allies and advocates for their particular interests. The District Management Team may seek the help of the CHC in its battles for extra funds with the AHA; surgeons may want the backing of the CHC in their struggle for new operating theatres, and so on. To this extent CHCs may, paradoxically become the voice of particular producer interests. Again, it would be wrong to imply that the producer interests necessarily clashes with the consumer interest; it is just as much in the interests of patients to have a good dermatology service as in those of the consultant concerned. But, clearly, the result could be that CHCs will come to share the priorities of those who, inescapably, see only the failings in their own particular sector of the NHS and do not perceive the larger pattern of needs and demands.

One possible outcome of setting up CHCs might, therefore, be to create a pressure group for more expenditure on the NHS while also making it more difficult to redistribute resources from one part of the country to another, or from one service to another, by cutting existing allocations [21]. As a result of setting up CHCs, a new kind of collective district patriotism may be created in opposition to national policies; the Government may have created extra pressures for spending just at the time when its capacity to satisfy it has shrunk [22]. Does this appear to be happening? To answer this question, the next section examines the activities of CHCs in their first year for what these tell us about their preoccupations and concerns.

Actions and reactions

Anyone coming to the annual reports of the Community Health Councils expecting to read an unrelieved litany of complaints about the state of the National Health Service would be disappointed. In line with the generally favourable assessment of health services made by individual CHC members, analysed in the previous chapter, there are some councils which explicitly proclaim their satisfaction:

> "Our Health Service is not perfect, but those who work in it should perhaps be aware of the British habit of self-denigration. In spite of its imperfections the experience of our Community Health Council... has revealed a system of health care which compares extremely well with any offered elsewhere... It is tempting for an organisation like ours to suggest major improvements regardless of cost but this would be a foolish pursuit if little or no likelihood existed for such a project being implemented". (Exeter)

Others are more critical and more demanding. The tendency of CHCs to involve themselves in local campaigns to persuade the Government to provide funds to build a new hospital has already been illustrated. Nor is this surprising since the first year of CHCs coincided with a period of economic stringency when the Government was cutting back its capital investment plans for the NHS, which meant that many long-delayed and much-promised building projects were shelved yet again to the fury and frustration of staff and consumers alike. Again, there is no problem in finding examples of special pleading for more funds, even from areas with statistically above-average provision of resources:

"There is a strong case to be made for the East End of London being designated a 'priority area' for health care. The fabric of most of the hospitals is old and unsuited to modern medical care. The health statistics compare unfavourably with national averages. There is a chronic shortage of staff, particularly para-medical staff...". (City and Hackney)

To a degree, such protests and pleas may primarily be an exercise in expressive politics: a ritual dance performed not in the hope of persuading the heavens to send down gifts but to provide a ceremonial outlet for the frustrations of the local population. It allows CHCs to put on an aggressive performance — and thus to demonstrate to the local population that they are doing a good job — without alienating NHS professionals and administrators, who may well welcome such evidence of popular demand for extra staff, facilities or buildings. To make this point is not to denigrate the CHCs: rituals are important in politics, and the existence of a community voice in health matters may in itself bring satisfaction even if it does not produce any direct rewards.[23].

This interpretation is strengthened by what the CHCs did, as distinct from what they said. When it came to the point — when they actually had the opportunity to block moves which reduced local facilities — they turned out to be less militant than their words might suggest. With rare exceptions they accepted, without much demur, proposals for closing down hospitals and wards: a pattern which is all the more interesting since this is one of the few areas of activity where CHCs actually have some power, even it it is only the power of delay. If they object to closures or changes of use, the local health authority cannot override them without first getting approval of the Secretary of State.

So far, then, the result of introducing CHCs has been less to block change than to make the process of achieving it more time-consuming. The process of consultation in the NHS, before changes can be made, is in any case extremely cumbersome[24]. Staff interests, local authorities and others have to be involved, and the CHCs have added a further layer of complexity. For example, in the case of one maternity unit, a 1972 decision to close it was still being argued over and reviewed at the beginning of 197[25]. This case is especially interesting, since two Community Health Councils were at odds with each other. One supported the proposal for closure, while the other opposed it: a warning against assuming that the community interest is indivisible and homogeneous. In this particular instance, the two CHCs were representing the conflicting interests of two geographical populations: a pattern only too likely to recur when health facilities are being closed or re-sited, since different populations will be affected in different ways by such changes.

Delay in implementing decisions to close down expensively under-utilised health service facilities may, naturally, impose costs on the NHS. And there is some evidence that CHCs themselves are beginning to take the initiative in suggesting closures:

> "Owing to the current fall in birth rate, the Princess Beatrice is now under-used. This is an expensive building to maintain for an average of 40 patients at a time. We feel that the use of this building should be urgently reviewed. Although the birth rate may rise again, there are too many obstetric beds in Central London for the current demand, and we would question if it is justified to maintain this unit for teaching purposes only." (South Kensington, Chelsea and Westminster)

It would be dangerous to predict the future behaviour of CHCs in this respect on the basis of their first year record. Many of the proposals for closures and change of use were already in the pipe-line and CHCs, as they themselves frequently pointed out, felt that they had no option but to agree to the inevitable. Such acquiescence may not endure. Further, there is some evidence that CHCs vary in their attitudes according to the service concerned. The willingness to close maternity units, for example, is what might be expected from the low priority accorded by CHC members to this service. But a general reluctance to agree to the closure of facilities used by the whole population, in line with the higher priority given to services to ordinary and acutely ill patients, is illustrated by the following quotation:

> "The closure of the Bexhill Hospital Casualty Department was the subject of fierce debate and feeling among many residents, particularly because of the high proportion of elderly people in the area for whom travelling to the Royal East Sussex Hospital for first aid treatment is difficult. The Community Health Council, whilst appreciating that it might prove impracticable to restore full services at the Casualty Department of Bexhill Hospital, recognised the hardship and inconvenience caused by its total closure and supported the many organisations and inhabitants of Bexhill in their campaign to secure simple first aid treatment at Bexhill Hospital and sought a meeting with the Area Health Authority... The outcome, after consideration of a number of options, was that the Casualty Department at Bexhill should

remain closed, but that the provision of health centre facilities should be vigorously pursued". (Hastings)

So it is difficult to be sure how CHCs will, in future, react to the re-deployment of health service resources, if this means cutting local services. But the evidence suggests that it is unlikely to be a simply reflex reaction of outright opposition.

If the CHCs add to the pressures for more resources to be devoted to the NHS (or more likely, given the current economic climate, make it more difficult to cut back the growth in spending) it may be for rather different reasons. It is because their day to day activities drag out into the open, and give visibility to specific inadequacies in the provision of services: because they create an active awareness of deficiencies which otherwise tend to be accepted with passive and perhaps fatalistic acquiescence.

Most CHCs, as already noted, launched into their first year with an intensive round of visits to NHS facilities: whether this was a once-and-for-all exercise in self-education or will become part of an on-going routine, remains to be seen — and no doubt CHCs will continue to vary in their practices. Many reports are dominated by the response of the members to what they saw:

"**Royal Infirmary:** the original building dates from 1797 and in spite of much upgrading continues to evoke the response, fast becoming a cliche, that it attempts to practise 20th century medicine in an 18th century building. Its 450 beds provide for most of the main specialities... On Ward 19 and 20, though upgrading had occurred as far as internal decorations were concerned, the toilet accommodation was appalling with two toilets and one bathroom for upward of 20 women on one floor and a similar situation for men on another... Patients' beds were far too close together. There was no day-room facility... A visit to the hospital kitchen revealed some of the difficulties encountered in providing adequate and suitable catering facilities for patients and staff... Kitchen staff had to work below ground and with little natural light coming in. In bad weather the kitchen was often flooded and the lack of proper ventilation meant that food was often prepared and awaited distribution in very high temperatures". (Southern Sheffield)

"We feel our Health District must be unique in having an Accident & Emergency Centre at Pembury Hospital which has a corridor where two stretcher-trolleys cannot pass, serving Examination/Resuscitation rooms in which it is not possible to accommodate a patient together with a Resuscitation Team and its gear at one and the same time... orthopaedic patients requiring X-rays of some magnitude have to be trundled out in their beds on to the main hospital roadway and dodging the traffic are pushed up a one in three tarmac slope to the X-ray Department. This is an interesting experience for a patient strung round with gantrys and pulleys and requires porters of considerable strength". (Tunbridge Wells)

"Pavilion 12 was a large geriatric block, well over 100 years old containing three wards. The Hospital Authories had long been worried at the condition of the Pavilion and had in 1974 been successful in progressing a scheme for its up-grading... However, in February 1975 the financial crisis which had by then hit the Health Service appeared to have resulted in this scheme's postponement. At around this time, the Community Health Council's Geriatric Study Group visited the Pavilion... They were appalled by what they saw and immediately put their weight behind the District's case for the reinstatement of the scheme as an immediate priority". (South Manchester)

Some CHCs went further still. In one report, a model of its kind, the CHC analysed in detail the extent to which facilities at one particular hospital fell short of nationally laid down standards [26]:

"In hospitals with over 100 beds the minimum standard for kitchen staff is 1 per 45 persons fed, and 20% of the staff should be in supervisory grades. On 30th September 1974 the ratio at St. Bernard's was 1 staff to 88 persons fed and 13% of the staff were in supervisory grades... The circular states that 'all patients should be encouraged to purchase and wear their own clothes' ... at the end of last year 898 patients did not have a full range of clothing for their sole personal use... 'The aim should be for each patient to have a programme of occupation or rehabilitation specially adapted to his or her own individual needs'. When occupational activities were monitored on the first working day in November last year, 801 patients were not participating..." (Ealing)

These quotations suggest a number of conclusions. The first is that CHCs are not uncovering new information. Their role mostly appears to be to underline information which is available both to AHA members and administrators, and to give it a new salience. The second is that they are usually supporting, rather than threatening, the professionals. But criticism of conditions can easily spill over into criticism of the way in which professionals work as shown by the following comments by a CHC member following an inspection of a children's ward:

"Compared to a number of residential schools, I have recently visited I would say that the physical comforts were superior but the overall atmosphere depressing in view of the immense amount of money which had been spent. Beautiful toys were suspended from the ceilings well out of reach of the children... I was not happy to see the sister and two other nurses in one ward sitting down feeding the children from behind and above — so that the child could not see what was on his plate... I would suggest that further training might also be envisaged for the large number of immigrant nurses..." (North Camden)

So perhaps the third general conclusion to be drawn is that representing the consumer will involve impinging on issues which have hitherto been the reserve of management and professionals. If it is in the interests of the consumers to have improved standards, then inescapably the CHCs will be drawn into raising matters which have hitherto been the prerogatives of health care producers — perhaps invoking alternative professional conceptions of how things ought to be done.

The logic of such a development is simple. Since CHCs will always be told that the resources required to provide the improved services they want are not available, they will be drawn into making proposals for the better use of existing resources. And this means, in effect, challenging management decisions not so much from the consumer's point of view but from a more general public interest or commonsense concern with the efficient use of resources. Thus one CHC opposed the AHA's capital investment programme on the following grounds:

"**Leasowe Hospital:** proposed new entrance and car park £40,000. Reasons:— a) There is already an adequate car park at the rear of the hospital. b) A simple entrance would suffice to allow access of a Fire Engine...

St. James' Hospital: proposal to widen existing main entrance, £5,000. Reasons:— a) The present entrance is reasonable... b) The hospital is not a busy one... c) The entrance could be cheaply widened by the removal of the wrought iron pedestrian gateway". (North Wirral)

Local knowledge, this illustration suggests, may provide a new perspective on management decisions.

Much of the work of CHCs is concerned with the small change of life and work within the NHS. One CHC is worried about inadequate alarm bell system for patients, unsuitable toilets in hospitals for the handicapped, badly designed beds — "Some nurses have commented on the back trouble caused by beds of wrong heights". (Norwich). Another recommends that the ventilation and seating should be improved in the casualty department, that double sinks should be provided in the kitchens, that the nurses' quarters needed improvements, that bins for disposable milk bottles should be provided and that walls required repainting. (Havering). Yet a third comments on the lack of curtain screening round beds, on the shortage of domestic staff, defective heating systems and the failure to use three acres of land surrounding a hospital to grow vegetables. (Isle of Wight). Like a recurring refrain, there is a repeated emphasis on the shortage of lavatories, and similar deficiencies in the basics of hospital care; interestingly, too, many CHCs clearly identify the welfare of the consumer with the welfare of the staff, and frequently propose improvements designed to help the latter — as by providing creches or better transport for nurses. All this may seem very different from the overwhelming stress put by CHC members on their planning role, in reply to our questionnaire. And it suggests that many CHC members are largely concerned with the amenity aspects of the patient's life — how best to deal with the minor but niggling problems that can be created by lack of thought or lack of basic facilities. In this, the CHC members once more appear to reflect accurately the concerns of the consumers; surveys of patient opinion indicate that this is precisely the area of greatest dissatisfaction [27]. Planning and priorities may be the appropriate vocabulary for circulars; bed-pans and hot meals are what matters to most patients for most of the time.

To try to quantify these CHC activities would, as indicated at the beginning of this chapter, convey only a misleading impression of precision. But, impressionistically, a majority of CHCs seem most concerned about services for the elderly, in line with what would be expected from the views of individual members. Beyond that, it would be dangerous to draw any conclusions from the first set of reports about the extent to which CHCs have concentrated their attention on particular client groups.

But some specific concerns do emerge emphatically from the annual reports. There is, for example, considerable interest in the accessibility of health service facilities, and problems associated with the siting of hospitals and GP practices. This takes a variety of forms:

> "The Council has become aware of the need to provide accommodation for relatives of patients in the District's hospitals, many of whom have to travel long distances to be with those that are seriously ill. One of its

earliest recommendations therefore was for the provision of additional overnight facilities for these visitors". (Bristol)

"It is recognised that there is a national tendency to concentrate family doctor services in group practices operating from purpose built premises, and the CHC appreciates the benefits of this trend. Notwithstanding this, it must be accepted that the NHS authorities have a duty to provide health services which are reasonably accessible to the public". (Blackburn)

These quotations also underline a further problem faced by CHCs: that of confining their attention to what is ostensibly their parish — the health service. Since the accessibility of NHS services may depend as much on the policies being pursued about transport as on decisions taken by health service authorities, CHCs find themselves implicitly extending their terms of reference. Similarly, the complementarity of health and personal social services is a cliche of policy making: one of the reasons for putting half the membership of CHCs into the gift of local authorities was precisely in order to strengthen such co-operation. But the logic of this is that the CHCs ought to be paying almost as much attention to the relevant local authority services as to those of the NHS, particularly when it comes to community support for the elderly or the mentally handicapped. And this can cause difficulties:

"It is vital to the effective functioning of a Community Health Council that the Health Authorities have a statutory obligation to consult it. It is a weakness of our relationship with local authorities that there is no parallel obligation in their case... In the circumstances, the Community Health Council feels there is a deficiency in the present structure which needs to be met if the CHC is to make any effective contribution...". (Great Yarmouth and Waveney)

Even within the NHS the activities of the CHCs have underlined the problems which may be caused by administrative demarcation lines. Among the preoccupations of many CHCs, inevitably, is general practice:

"Of all the services provided by the National Health Service, the Family Doctor Service is the one that is causing the most concern to the CHC, and we intend to continue to look into and comment upon the services provided by family doctors". (Mansfield and Newark)

"There is public unease about the anonymity, size and location of health centres, which are often deemed to be for the convenience of doctors but not of the patients; about doctors prescribing without consultation and about receptionists fobbing off patients who want to consult..." (Bolton)

But general practice is very much an autonomous enclave within the reorganised NHS [28] : the service is administered by Family Practitioner Committees and GPs, in contrast to hospital doctors, are independent contractors. So while CHCs have a statutory right to visit hospitals, this does not apply to the premises of GPs. The result is that CHCs may find themselves blocked when their activities extend into the realm of general practice:

> "We were concerned to receive a memorandum from the Avon Family Practitioner Committee which... stated that the FPC is generally not prepared to respond to approaches from CHCs concerning doctors' practice arrangements 'since
>
> a) the arrangements have been made to the satisfaction of the Family Practitioner Committee, and
>
> b) they have not resulted in any criticism by individual patients — if they had, a statutory enquiry would have taken place and any necessary adjustments would have been made'.
>
> The implication of this memorandum is most disturbing to us since it seems that the FPC is seeking to tell CHCs what they may or may not do. We surely have the right to challenge even arrangements which have the approval of the FPC". (Weston)

This particular example of conflict is unusual though not unique; in many instances, CHCs and FPCs appear to have come to an amicable working arrangement. But it does illustrate the scope for friction created when the logic of looking at patient care from the consumer's point of view parts company from the logic of administrative arrangements.

In the case of the family practitioner service, there is at least well-established — if not invariably smooth-working — machinery for dealing with complaints from the public [29] . But even this, as the Davies Committee pointed out [30] , does not exist in the rest of the NHS. So it is not surprising that there was some initial apprehension among Ministers and civil servants lest CHCs should concentrate excessively on complaints. This partly helps to explain the emphasis, in the notes of guidance given to CHC members, on the constructive aspects of their work and the warning about what they should and should not do about complaints: [31]

> "The investigation of individual complaints will be a matter for the health authority and its staff or (where appropriate) for the Health

Commissioner or Service Committee but Community Health Councils will be able, without prejudging the merits of individual complaints or seeking out the facts, to give advice, on request, on how and where to lodge a complaint and to act as a 'patient's friend' when needed"

A few CHCs were puzzled as to how to interpret this somewhat tortuous language. Some, however, adopted an active policy of encouraging the public to bring their complaints to the CHC: this was seen as yet another way of establishing closer links with the community and perhaps also as a way of ensuring that the work of the CHC would receive attention from the local media. But direct clashes with the health authorities, arising out of individual cases, appear to have been rare. One CHC took up the case of a mentally handicapped person who died in hospital as the result of scalds, where "at the inquest no approach was made to the parents by anybody from the hospital, the District Management Team or the Area Health Authority, either to offer sympathy or to explain what further investigation could be made" (Ealing); another enlisted the local MP in a campaign to find a place for a mentally handicapped boy in a special-care hostel (Huddersfield). For the most part, the sections of the reports dealing with complaints serve chiefly to illustrate the elasticity, ambiguity and vagueness of the word itself. This is why, although many reports give figures of complaints, it would be futile to try to analyse the total since so many disparate items feature under this heading and different CHCs use different definitions.

Some CHCs attempt to distinguish between enquiries and complaints. But one man's enquiry about where to get a particular service may be another man's complaint about the inadequacy of existing services, and the dividing line is often blurred. Again, one CHC (East Dorset) distinguishes between "grumbles, comments and suggestions", on the one hand, and "protests, grievances and accusations", on the other, but most CHCs do not attempt such a sophisticated break-down. Characteristic of the very miscellaneous business done by CHCs are the following extracts from one council's list of matters dealt with:

"Telephone call from patient complaining that he had been refused general medical examination by GP...

Call from patient... who was concerned that he was going to be discharged without suitable accommodation to go to...

Letter from College of Further Education complaining of breakdown in referral services for student who had reached crisis point...

> Call at office from elderly lady who wished to discuss what she felt were the shortcomings of the Health Service, such as provision of spectacles and dentistry for old people. She had no specific complaint...
>
> Letter from lady complaining that she had inadequate supervision while taking the pill...". (South Camden)

The same point is made by another CHC's illustration of the kinds of queries received:

> "Mrs. G. Requesting information on head lice...
>
> Mrs. N. Worried about E.S.N. son (early 30's, living at home) in event of parents' death...
>
> Mr. S. Requesting advice on vasectomy...". (North Hammersmith)

These examples suggest that CHCs are largely, though not exclusively, dealing with inquiries or complaints about the availability of services. In contrast, for example, to the Health Commissioner [32] or to the formal machinery for dealing with complaints, they are dealing not so much with maladministration in the delivery and organisation of services, as with inadequacies in the provision of services. The two are, of course, not always easy to separate in practice — and when a particular service is unavailable to the patient, it may be either because existing resources are being badly deployed or because the existing level of provision is quite simply insufficient. But to make the distinction is also to suggest that the CHCs will have a continuing role even if the NHS machinery for dealing with complaints is made more accessible and given greater scope, in line with the recommendations of the Davies Committee. Additionally, CHCs appear to be playing a very considerable role in dispensing comfort, re-assurance and advice to worried or lonely people, whose complaints may represent less a criticism of the NHS than a plea for someone to take an interest in their problems. This seems to be one of the informal functions both of shop-front offices run by CHCs and of the evening "surgeries" which some of them have organised. It could well turn out that the CHCs will be playing a role for which they were never designed, but where their emergence on the scene has revealed a hitherto unfilled gap — supporting, rather than representing, the consumer of health services.

What difference have the CHCs made?

So far the discussion of the first year's record of the CHCs has, very deliberately, avoided the one question which is probably foremost in the minds of most readers. What difference have CHCs made to the way in which the National Health Service operates? This is partly, as indicated in the introduction, because the time-span involved is too short. CHCs have not been in existence long enough to make a significant impact. But, more fundamentally, it is because the question itself is strictly unanswerable within the limits of our research strategy and the information available about the operations of the National Health Service.

The point can simply be illustrated by the report of one CHC which introduces its "success stories" as follows:

> "Frequently, of course, the Area Health Authority have already decided to make the improvements recommended by the Council but the following improvements have been carried out after recommendations were made by the Council...". (Cornwall)

The report then lists such items as "further improvement of the meals service at St. Lawrence's hospital ... Re-surfacing of the entrance drive at Tehidy hospital ... Improvements have been made in the arrangements for the transport and care of elderly patients from Barncoose hospital ... Elimination of draught through the external double doors to the kitchen and providing additional car parking space at Treliske ..." and so on. And, no doubt, there would be little difficulty in finding similar examples of action following CHC recommendations, if only on small scale matters, elsewhere in the country. But all this might indicate is that when CHCs push at an open door, then it swings open. Listing such success stories might create an entirely misleading impression of power and influence.

But just to concentrate on those changes of policy which follow after a head-on collision between CHCs and health authorities would be equally misleading. For this is to ignore the possibility that the impact of CHCs might be greatest when health authorities act pre-emptively to avoid a conflict with them: the "rule of anticipated reactions" [33], which suggests that the influence of representative bodies can often be best measured by the pains taken by executives to anticipate their views in order to prevent any clash. Account would have to be taken not only of what is done by health authorities but also what is not done: for instance, it could well be that some hospitals might not be closed because the District Management Teams concerned were not prepared to put their hands into the hornet's nest of CHC opposition.

Above all, there is the risk of defining the success or failure of CHCs in narrow but measurable terms — so many complaints successfully handled, so many rules successfully changed, so many extra lavatories installed etc. — while neglecting what may be more important dimensions. For example, if their existence leads to changes in the style of health service administration — in the way in which administrators and professionals approach and perceive their task — then the introduction of CHCs will have made a major difference to the NHS. So the next, and concluding chapter examines the role of the CHC from this wider perspective and considers what policy implications can be drawn from the experience so far.

1 For a general discussion see, apart from Pitkin (op.cit), A.H. Birch *Representation* Macmillan 1971. More specifically, on the distinction between different representative roles, see J.C. Wahlke, H. Eulau, W. Buchanan and L. Ferguson *The Legislative system: explorations in legislative behaviour* J. Wiley & Sons 1962.

2 Four case studies of individual CHCs — Anglesey, Bath, North-West Kensington, Chelsea and Westminster and Wigan — are being published as a separate Working Paper, edited by Janet Lewis. In addition, our analysis has been enriched by conversations with CHC secretaries and members met at seminars, conferences and elsewhere.

3 The most recent of these, shows that 80 out of the 100 people interviewed were not aware of the existence or functions of Community Health Councils. See, Frada Eskin and Peter Newton 'Public ignorance of the health service' *Health and Social Services Journal* 10 April 1976.

4 Consumer Council *Consumer Consultative Machinery in the Nationalised Industries* HMSO 1968.

5 Commission on the Constitution Research Papers No.7 *Devolution and other aspects of Government: an attitudes survey* HMSO 1973 pp.9/10.

6 Committee on the Management of Local Government Vol.5 *Local government administration in England and Wales* HMSO 1967 See, Chapter 17.

7 Rudolf Klein *Notes towards a theory of patient involvement.* Working Paper Centre for Studies in Social Policy 1975.

8 The literature on professionalism is vast. But the following are particularly relevant: Terence J. Johnson *Professions and Power* Macmillan 1972; Eliot Freidson *Professional Dominance* Atherton Press 1970; Everett Hughes *Men and their work* The Free Press 1958.

9 Joint Consultants Committee 'Report of proceedings' *British Medical Journal* 8 November 1975.

10 Albert Spanswick 'NHS — reorganisation or disorganisation?" *Health Services* April 1975.

11 Willis J. Goudy and Robert O. Richards 'Citizens, bureaucrats and legitimate authority: some unanticipated consequence within the administration of social action programme' *Midwest Review of Public Administration* Vol.8 No.5. July 1974.

12 For a survey of the literature and a critical analysis of the concept, see Kenneth John Meier 'Representative bureaucracy: an empirical analysis' *American Political Science Review* Vol. LXIX No.2. June 1975. Also, Kenneth Kernaghan 'Responsible public bureaucracy: a rationale and a framework for analysis' *Canadian Public Administration* Vol.16 No.4. Winter 1973.

13 Royal Commission on Local Government in England Research Studies No.9. *Community Attitudes Survey: England* HMSO 1969 Table 107.

14 *A review of the management of the reorganised NHS* Association of Chief Administrators of Health Authorities, 1976.

15 R.G.S. Brown, S. Griffin and S.C. Haywood *New bottles: old wine?* University of Hull 1975.

16 Department of Health and Social Security *Management Arrangements for the reorganised National Health Service* HMSO 1972. But as late as 1975, the DHSS was still discussing the future introduction of the planning system. See DHSS circular *National Health Service Planning Systems* HSC (IS) 126 March 1975.

17 *Report of the Committee of Inquiry, held at Memorial Hospital, Darlington* Northern Regional Health Authority 1976.

18 Rudolf Klein and Phoebe Hall *Caring for quality in the caring services* Bedford Square Press 1973. For the change in name and scope, see DHSS circular *The Health Advisory Service* HC (76)21 April 1976.

19 Report of Committee of Enquiry *St. Augustine's Hospital, Chartham, Canterbury* South East Thames Regional Health Authority, 1976.

20 Department of Health and Social Security. Letter to administrators of RHAs and AHAs *Communication of HAS reports to CHCs* 10 June 1975.

21 For current spending targets, see Department of Health and Social Security circular *NHS planning system: DHSS planning guidelines for 1976/7* HC(76) 29 May 1976. Note the emphasis in this on the need for a "searching review" of existing services so that "those services which are relatively well-provided with facilities and staff can yield resources to those which are under-developed".

22 Rudolf Klein, Martin Buxton and Quentin Outram *Constraints and choices* Centre for Studies in Social Policy 1976.

23 Murray Edelman *The symbolic uses of politics* University of Illinois 1964.

24 Rudolf Klein 'A policy for a change' *British Medical Journal* 7 February 1976.

25 Agenda for meeting of the North East Thames Regional Health Authority, 26 January 1976.

26 Department of Health and Social Security circular *Minimum standards in hospitals for the mentally ill* DS86/72 March 1972.

27 Winifred Raphael *Patients and their hospitals* King Edward's Hospital Fund for London 1969; Winifred Raphael and Valerie Peers *Psychiatric hospitals viewed by their patients* King Edward's Hospital Fund for London 1972.

28 Rudolf Klein 'NHS Reorganisation: the politics of the second best' *The Lancet* 26 August 1972.

29 Rudolf Klein *Complaints against doctors* Charles Knight 1973.

30 *Report of the Committee on Hospital Complaints Procedure* HMSO 1973.

31 Department of Health and Social Security circular *Community Health Councils* HRC (74)4 January 1974.

32 Rudolf Klein 'The Health Commissioner' *The Lancet* 26 February 1972.

33 Carl J. Friedrich *Constitutional government and democracy* Ginn and Company 1946.

5

Policy implications and options

If Community Health Councils did not exist, would it be necessary to invent them? In one sense, the question answers itself. CHCs were largely devised, as we saw in the first chapter, for presentational reasons. They are, therefore, a political necessity. No Government, whether Labour or Conservative, could get rid of them without appearing to be cocking a snook at democracy, participation and consumerism — vague but vogue terms all in the rhetoric of political argument and powerfully resonant in their appeal. For any Minister to express scepticism about this trinity is to risk much the same fate which would have overtaken Victorian politicians who publicly professed doubts about the existence of the Holy Family: agnosticism on these questions is best left to consenting adults meeting in private.

Such political considerations should not be dismissed out of hand. The symbolic role of CHCs — as a reminder that certain broad values are cherished in principle by society — is important in its own right. But, before turning to an analysis of future options for policy-making, this chapter looks at CHCs from a somewhat different perspective. If it had not been politically expedient to create Community Health Councils, we ask in effect, would it still have been desirable to do so?

The National Health Service is a peculiar sort of organisation. In the first place, it is a virtual monopoly: the private sector is both small and specialised [1]. Secondly, the services provided by the NHS are uniquely heterogeneous. There is no currency in which its activities can be summed up at the end of the year in the way the nationalised industries, for example, can turn in a profit-and-loss account; the problems of both political and administrative control are exceptionally unyielding. Since there is no way of drawing up a balance sheet, control tends to take the form of detailed scrutiny. Thirdly, to add to these difficulties, the delivery of services in the NHS is the responsibility of professionals who see themselves accountable for the quality of their performance only to their fellow professionals[2]. If anyone were to ask whether the NHS was providing a better service in 1976 than in 1966, there would be a stunned silence. No one is either equipped or charged with carrying out such an assessment, and no one knows whether overall standards are rising or falling — or what criteria should be applied in assessing them [3].

In these circumstances, there is a positive argument for creating some machinery for encouraging actively the flow of consumer views, as a form of customer audit of the services being provided. This is not to deny that there are already means by which dissatisfied NHS customers can register their views: by approaching MPs or using the complaints machinery, although remarkably few do so [4]. Such individual approaches are expensive in time and require considerable commitment: by definition, they will provide a biased impression. Hence the case for an institution like the CHC which makes it easier and cheaper for individuals or groups to make their opinions, grievances or protests heard. In other words, the justification for CHCs may be less that they represent the public or the community (whatever that may mean) but that they provide a ready-made platform for those who wish to speak. Additionally, CHCs may well be able to abstract general issues from personal problems.

Alternative strategies for eliciting consumer preferences are, of course, conceivable. Instead of making it easier for people to voice their views, it might be possible to facilitate their exit [5]. They could be encouraged to vote with their feet by changing their consultant or their GP so that those hospitals or practices which offer an unsatisfactory service, from the consumer's point of view, simply lost their custom. Unfortunately the trend within the NHS is in precisely the opposite direction: the concentration of resources — into health centres, for example — is making it more difficult to exercise choice within the NHS. To reverse this trend, and to adopt a policy of deliberately encouraging more choice within the NHS, would imply a willingness to invest more resources and thus create some slack in the system.

There still remains the option of exit from the NHS into the private sector. But the opportunities for exercising this option are limited by the geographical distribution of private practice, by the fact that only a limited range of facilities are available and by the differential ability of people to afford the fees, even with the aid of insurance. To increase the scope for exit from the NHS would mean deliberately encouraging the growth of the private sector, perhaps by introducing a system of vouchers [6] which might enable more people to use it.

But if it is assumed that the NHS will remain a near-monopoly in the provision of health care for the foreseeable future, and that consequently the option of exit will be available only to a minority, then it is difficult to resist the argument for facilitating voice. It may be said, to return to an earlier argument, that the consumer is incapable of rational choice anyway, since he or she is not equipped to assess the professional competence of the service providers: so why make it easier to air views which are not entitled to respect? But this, like the alternative model of the consumer as an omniscient shopper, is over-simplified. There are areas of health care where the consumer, by the very fact of being a consumer, does know better than the professional provider or planner. He knows better about the quality of care even if he may know less about the quality of cure. He certainly is better able to tell whether health facilities are conveniently sited or whether the manners of health professionals are welcoming or coldly dictatorial. If the professional's knowledge is less than total, so is the consumer's ignorance. They are experts about entirely different aspects of a health care system and the problem in decision-making about the allocation and use of resources lies precisely in how best to balance demands reflecting consumer and professional perspectives. All such decisions are therefore bound to be political in the sense of judgments about priorities in a situation where the costs and benefits are measured in values rather than money.

In this context, the justification for an institution like the CHC lies precisely in the fact that it has widened the political arena within which discussions about the allocation and use of NHS resources take place. It has brought onto the stage a new set of political actors who, in the past, were left lurking in the wings of the theatre or hanging about the stage-door. And while individual consumers have only a limited interest in agitating for improved conditions — since they themselves may not benefit from any changes that may result and may even suffer retaliation — consumers collectively have an interest that such campaigns should be pursued and in the creation of bodies like CHCs which take over the costs involved and invest the required effort on their behalf [7]. In other words, the CHC is the good citizen institutionalised and financed out of public funds in order to be able to perform the role which the individual good citizen may not be able or willing to carry out in practice.

But institutionalising voice is not the same thing as ensuring that anyone will listen to the resulting sounds. It may have an expressive function, but it will not necessarily be an effective one. There is a danger that the means will be confused with the aims of policy. Democracy is as much about the way things are done as about formal institutions,[8] about the accessibility, responsiveness and openness of administrative systems as well as about setting up new machinery for conveying the views of consumers. If the machinery is simply going to grind away in a void, then the result may merely be to increase frustration.

This is why it is essential to consider not only the general case for having an institution like the CHC but also the specific circumstances which are calculated to make it effective, and this we do in the subsequent sections of this chapter which deal with particular policy options. But there is one further general point to be made, since it will colour the rest of the discussion. This is that all public and private organisations — and not just the British NHS or the British civil service — develop defensive techniques for filtering out disturbing noises[9]. Accessibility, responsiveness and openness cannot be taken for granted; if they could, there would not have been so much fuss in Britain and elsewhere[10] in recent years about ways of encouraging such administrative qualities. Hence the case for deliberately changing the structure of incentives, by introducing a new institution like the CHC, which increases the costs to administrators of ignoring outside views and pressures.

Leaving aside these general considerations for having an institution like the CHC, which spring from the nature of public service monopolies, there is a reinforcing argument based on the particular circumstances of the British NHS. Increasingly, the National Health Service is being run on syndicalist lines[11], to an extent which was perhaps not foreseen at the time of reorganisation. Since the start of the NHS, the medical profession has had a strong presence on all health authorities. This presence was given statutory recognition under reorganisation and extended to the nursing profession. And with the subsequent decision of the 1974 Labour Government to include two members elected by trade unions on each Area Health Authority — a move which will almost certainly generate pressure from the medical and nursing professions to elect their own representatives — another, major step was taken towards workers' control. The case for regarding the NHS as a syndicalist organisation could be strengthened still further by looking at decision-making at the district level, where a system of consensus management and an elaborate machinery of consultation means that health service workers exert a very large measure of influence.

Almost by accident, therefore, the NHS seems to be in the process of becoming the first of the "self-governing guilds" which were proposed by G.D.H. Cole [12] in the 'twenties as the best way of running public services. But this brand of syndicalist theory also assumed that if associations of workers took control of public (and other) services, then — to hold the balance — there should be corresponding associations of consumers. Cole and the Guild Socialists, for example, argued for local Health Councils, as well as for other Councils to represent the interests of consumers in education and other services. They accepted that the majority of people might be uninterested but argued that "functional representation, with the election of *ad hoc* authorities, very properly gives those who do want something and do take an interest the best opportunity of making their voice heard".

This theory is worth recalling because of its recognition that the development of producer-power implies also the development of a countervailing consumer-power: here, in a sense, is the historical root of the Community Health Council — even though it may not be recognised as such by those who reinvented it in the 'seventies. The theory is rather less helpful, unfortunately, in its detailed specifications. Cole took a somewhat Panglossian view of the relationship between producer-Guilds and consumer-Councils: these would have "not an antagonistic but a co-operative and complementary relationship. The Councils would exist to make articulate the spiritual and physical demands of the people, and to co-operate with the various Guilds which would have entrusted to them the task of supplying these demands". He did not address himself to the problems caused by the basic asymmetry in the relationship: the fact that the Guilds would have command over resources while the Councils, seemingly, were to have no compensatory sanctions. All conflict was to be dissolved in mutual good-will.

So while all these considerations suggest that if Community Health Councils did not exist, it would be necessary to invent *some* institutional device for strengthening the consumer voice, they do not answer the question of whether the existing machinery is the most suitable that could be devised to meet the need. The following sections therefore examine the practical policy options in the light of these wider, theoretical arguments.

The case for doing nothing

Those who write about institutions tend to acquire a vested interest in advocating change: why, after all, should they laboriously identify and analyse problems if, at the end of the day, they conclude that nothing should be done about the strains or flaws revealed? Inventing what may be unnecessary proposals for reform is an occupational hazard which must be guarded against, and the first policy option which requires exposition is that of doing nothing and leaving the Community Health Councils exactly as they are or, at most, tinkering with minor details in their constitution.

There are two, quite separate kinds of arguments for the *status quo*. The first is to claim that Community Health Councils should be left alone because they have done a successful job: what might be called the strong case for doing nothing. The second is to argue that, since the NHS is only at the stage of convalescence after the trauma of reorganisation, the onus of proof must be on those who demand change, and that while CHCs may not have made much of a positive contribution, neither are they doing any harm: what might be called the weak case for continuing with the existing state of affairs.

On the evidence available so far, the weak case is more persuasive than the strong case. Not only is it too early to come to any firm conclusion about the success or otherwise of CHCs; more important still, as our analysis in the previous chapters have documented, there are a variety of different — and to some extent conflicting — ways of looking at their role and consequently of judging their performance. Further, if CHCs have not yet made any clear-cut impact in the service, this may be as much because of the general problems of engineering change in the National Health Service — which have perplexed and frustrated successive generations of Secretaries of State, civil servants and administrators — as because of any specific weakness in the constitution of the councils. Disappointment that the injection of CHCs appears to have done little to affect attitudes or policies may simply reflect unrealistic expectations about the potential for short-term change.

This said, it is important to try to imagine what the reorganised NHS would be like if there were no CHCs. There would be no band of inquisitive men and women going round hospitals and other facilities asking the occasional awkward question or looking at the small-change of patient comfort. There would be no one to argue the case for providing more information about what was happening in the NHS and pressing for a less introspective and more open style of decision-making. There would be no one to provide a platform for individuals or pressure groups — whether the rival fluoridation lobbies or the midwives seeking to exclude men from exercising their profession — who want to make their case heard or seek allies. There would be no institutionalised way of bringing official rhetoric about what is desirable face to face with the realities of what is happening locally.

If the accents in which CHCs speak are heavily middle-class this may — it is possible to argue — even be an advantage, since (to paraphrase Nye Bevan) generalising the best in the NHS probably can be safely translated to mean generalising the standards which the most demanding middle-class consumers expect for themselves. If democracy is about accessibility to the policy-making process, among many other things, then the very existence of CHCs represents an addition to the otherwise available opportunities, and is desirable as such.

But there is another side to this particular balance sheet. Although it would be difficult to maintain that CHCs do any harm, they certainly impose costs on the NHS. These cannot be reckoned merely in terms of the £3,000,000 or so — about 0.05% of the total NHS budget — allocated to them by the regional authorities to pay for their staff and offices. Nor can it be comprehensively measured even by including an allowance for the administrative costs generated by CHCs: the staff time devoted to dealing with their queries or demands for information. Possibly these administrative costs might double the total annual bill — which would still be an almost invisible proportion of all spending on health care.

More important, there are also frictional costs to be taken into account: extra pressures on already busy people, administrative timidity reinforced, policies deferred or not considered for fear of stirring up controversy, and so on. More open administration may also be slower administration. While it is popular to protest about the delays imposed by bureaucracy, and the difficulty of getting anyone in the NHS to make a decision, it is less fashionable to talk about the time lost as a result of the complex consultative process [13] . In addition, greater responsiveness to local demands could well mean providing expensive facilities which could be supplied more cheaply elsewhere.

To an extent, therefore, the view taken of CHCs must depend on the assessment made of the desirability and effectiveness of national planning. If it is thought that the overriding aim of the NHS must be to move towards a system of national priorities, reflecting decisions about how national resources can be used most efficiently, then CHCs can easily be seen as one further hurdle on what is already a formidable obstacle course. But, of course, it may well be thought that the central decision-makers are less than infallible: for example, in the 'sixties they were advocating giant hospitals, in the 'seventies they have discovered the advantages of much smaller nuclear hospitals [14]. Moreover, such concepts as the efficient use of resources are more ambiguous than often appears at first sight: the concentration of resources may be efficient from the point of view of producers but may be less so from the point of view of the consumers who spend the time and money travelling longer distances. So if the claims and advantages of national planning are viewed more sceptically, delay may even be seen as a beneficial device for saving the decision-makers from the consequences of their own mistakes by giving them time to correct course.

Overall, then, there would seem to be no compelling, overriding case for disturbing the NHS by amputating the Community Health Councils. But this is not to say that CHCs should be considered sacrosanct or inviolable if, in the next few years, a Government were to decide to change the present structure of the NHS for other reasons. In a changing NHS, there would also be scope for changes in the way the consumer interest is represented.

The case for integration

If there were a clear-cut consumer interest in the National Health Service opposed to a sharply defined producer interest, the gladiatorial model implied by reorganisation would be appropriate and there would be no reason to question the existing arrangements for institutionalising conflict by means of Community Health Councils. But in practice, as we have seen, it has proved impossible to maintain the fiction that a clear line can be drawn between representation and management. CHCs are increasingly being drawn into matters which would normally be defined as managerial: indeed they have been prodded in this direction by the Department of Health and Social Security. Many of them appear to see themselves as a kind of counter-management, making recommendations about the use of resources. What is more, most CHC members — to judge from their responses to our questionnaire — seem to think of themselves as making a constructive rather than a critical contribution.

So we come to the seemingly paradoxical conclusion that friction between consumer representatives and NHS managers and professionals stems not from a conflict of interest but from an overlap of interests. It is because the managers and professionals see themselves as responsible for making the plans that they resent the interference of CHCs and at times refuse information or access to the decision-making process. It is because many CHC members see themselves as part of the managerial and planning machinery that they resent lack of involvement in the policy-making process. It is because everyone thinks that he or she has the best interests of the patient at heart that there is argument about who really is the consumer's best friend.

One way out of this dilemma would be to abolish the Community Health Councils as free-standing institutions and incorporate them explicitly into the hierarchy of the NHS administrative structure. This would be to accept that the distinction drawn between the members of Area Health Authorities and of Community Health Councils — between the board of directors and the representatives of the public, as it were — was unrealistic in the first place and has been made unsustainable by the decision to increase the local authority membership of the AHAs and so create even more overlap between the two sets of bodies.

There are at least two policy options for integrating CHCs into the structure of the NHS. The first would be to dissolve them totally but incorporate that part of their membership which is not already represented — those nominated by voluntary organisations — in the Area Health Authorities. The main argument against this is that it would swell the size of AHAs, already inflated by the inclusion of more local authority and trade-union members, to bursting point. Additionally, the result would be to diminish the number of lay outsiders involved in the running of the NHS.

Alternatively , Community Health Councils could become the district committees of the AHAs: a return, in effect, to the proposals in Richard Crossman's 1970 Green Paper. In practice, some AHAs have already begun to set up sub-committees responsible for looking at services in individual districts. So there would be a persuasive case for formalising and building on this trend. While AHAs would continue to have overall managerial responsibility for policy, district committees could be charged with reporting on the delivery of services in their own community from the consumer's perspective. They would be generating the information about shortfalls and shortcomings which is the required raw material for management decisions. They would be explicitly involved in the processes leading up to policy decisions, even though they would not be formally responsible for them. In multi-district AHAs, at any rate, it should thus be possible to design complementary rather than conflicting — because overlapping — roles for authority and committee members.

The argument against this option is the same as the case against the original Crossman proposals: that, like the members of the defunct Hospital Mangement Committees, those serving on district committees might become too involved in the managerial processes and lose the capacity to act as the consumer's advocate. But, speculatively, there might be another way of trying to resolve the problem of preventing consumer representatives becoming frustrated through lack of access to the managerial processes and the authority members becoming too management-minded as a result of their involvement in the administrative processes. One of the present advantages of CHCs members over AHA members is that they have independent sources of information and advice: they are served by their own secretariat. In contrast, members of AHAs (like elected members of local authorities) are serviced by the very people whose activities they are monitoring: the officers of the authority. It may, therefore, be worth considering the possibility of providing an independent secretariat for both AHA and district committee members — should CHCs be incorporated into the managerial structure of the NHS — so as to make them both less dependent on the officers. In other words, the division would be less between officers and professionals at different levels — districts and AHAs [15] — and more between lay members and managers. Just as Ministers have increasingly recruited special advisers whose first loyalty is to them, rather than to the organisation, so members of NHS authorities and committees would have their own staff whose first loyalty would be to them rather than to the managerial hierarchy.

The case for strenthening "voice"

The case for incorporating CHCs into the administrative structure of the NHS rests on the assumption that the best way of resolving the tension between managerial and representative functions is to bring the two elements together in one organisation, and not to try to impose over-simple and artificial institutional models on the complex pattern of human behaviour. But if this option is rejected, there is an alternative approach. This starts from the assumption that the trouble about the gladiatorial theory of consumer representation is not that is has been proved wrong by events, but that it has never been tried in practice. When it came to applying the theory to CHCs, the nerves of Ministers and civil servants broke at the last fence. The prospect of institutionalised criticism proved too much. Hence the decision to give CHCs a more constructive —

which, in effect, was a more managerial — role; hence, too, the friction and frustration caused by overlapping interests and functions.

The solution would thus appear to be simple. It would be to return to first principles, withdraw the advice to CHCs to assess services and make constructive proposals, and instead instruct them firmly and unambiguously that their only role is to act as a platform for whichever individual consumer or interest groups want to make use of them. CHCs would be firmly identified as a collective community resource, charged with facilitating the expression of consumer views. Just as communities collectively provide pipe-lines for supplying water to their citizens, so they would be providing pipe-lines for transmitting messages to the NHS. The CHC would be seen not so much as the voice or spokesman of the community — a phrase which assumes that there is necessarily one common interest — as an instrument for making it easier for individuals or groups to make their voices heard.

This is an inadequate, because partial, view. It is to equate representation with communication. It leaves out of account the role of the CHC — stressed above — in exerting pressure to make sure that messages are not only transmitted but receive some attention. It is to neglect the possibility that, in some circumstances at any rate, there may be a collective community view on specific issues. It is to overlook the role of CHCs in representing those who cannot speak for themselves: the mentally handicapped, the senile and so on.

To make these points is to stress the importance of authority and perceived legitimacy: if CHCs are to speak effectively on behalf of the community or individuals and groups within it, then there must be a recognition that their members have a right to express views and to be heard. To some extent CHCs may acquire such authority because Ministers and civil servants listen to their views with respect and solicit their comments on national issues; even the appearance of influence may help to bring about the reality. But at least equally important, is the extent to which CHCs are regarded as being representative of their communities, and in what ways. If they are perceived to be representative (in one or other of the many meanings of the word), then their intervention will be felt as legitimate — even if resented — rather than merely being rejected as the meddlings of self-selected busy-bodies.

Indeed it might be argued that if the only object of the exercise were to elicit consumer opinions and preferences — as distinct from having a voice which can speak with authority on behalf of the consumer — then there are easier, and perhaps more accurate ways, of achieving this aim than by setting up CHCs. For example, it might be possible to have systematic surveys at both the local and the national level or to use other techniques for getting a picture of people's priorities: arguably these would reflect public attitudes more sensitively than the CHCs which, as we have seen, represent the views of people who are unrepresentative in their education, experience and commitment to voluntary or public service.

But representation has two aspects. The first is the characteristics of the representatives: a subject already explored in detail in Chapter 2. The other is the relationship between the representatives and the represented. The present method of selecting CHC members deliberately tries, as noted earlier, to make them unrepresentative in that it stresses that they owe a collective loyalty to the NHS rather than being individually accountable to the bodies which nominate them. This makes sense in the context of emphasising their quasi-managerial function. But if this concept were abandoned, there would be every reason for recognising CHC members as representatives in the full sense: that is, speaking for, and accountable to, their constituents. This point has been made strongly in connection with the consultative committees attached to the nationalised industries [16]:

> "... a true representative, whether of the consumer interest or any other interest, must by definition have a body of constitutents who have given him their confidence, by some formal voting procedure, and to whom he is responsible. It is the lack of responsibility to any constituency that vitiates the present arrangements for consumer 'representation'."

Following on from this, there flows the question of what the appropriate constituencies are. On this point, DHSS policy continues to hedge its bets as between stressing voluntary organisations concerned with special health service interests and those with other, perhaps wider interests [17]. Similarly, it continues to stress the importance of using the RHA nominees to ensure the presence of CHC members involved with immigrants and religious organisations, as well as trade-unions. To judge by our survey evidence about the membership of these various organisations, this concern is largely redundant. There would seem to be a strong case for allowing more self-selection, and allowing a vote in the nomination of CHC members to all voluntary organisations interested enough to wish to take part.

But this still assumes that the present system of nominating CHC members — one half by local authorities, one third by voluntary organisations and one-sixth by the RHAs — should be perpetuated. This is far from self-evident. There is, as yet, little evidence that the presence of local authority councillors creates greater co-operation between local government and the NHS, while there is convincing evidence that many of those deeply involved in local government work do not have time to spare for CHCs. Nor, on the whole, does our survey indicate that authority nominees contribute a distinctive style of perception or way of assessing services. This method of nomination appears to make only one measurable difference to the composition of CHCs: it increases the proportion of blue-collar workers, as we have seen. But it also strengthens their links with the political network.

A longer-term option, in these circumstances, might be to transfer the present local authority seats to the Neighbourhood Councils, if and when these develop [18]. These will represent the small "natural" communities of between 3,000 and 10,000 people whose size is most calculated to encourage citizen involvement; at the same time, precisely because their size is too small to allow them to run any services, there is every likelihood that they may not have enough to do to sustain interest in their activities. Involving them in the NHS might serve the double purpose of helping Neighbourhood Councils to survive, while at the same time providing a natural constituency for Community Health Councils. Where parish councils or community councils already exist, these could nominate CHC members should such a system be adopted.

To introduce the Neighbourhood Councils into the discussion of policy options for consumer involvement in the NHS is also to draw attention to a wider dilemma. This is that the technical logic of organising the delivery of health services does not necessarily coincide — and arguably is diametrically opposed to — the logic of inventing new forms of consumer representation. Opinions differ, and have changed over time, about the size of population required to sustain a comprehensive health care service centred on a district general hospital: the range is somewhere between 100,000 and 300,000. But whether the higher or lower figure is chosen as appropriate, this is a much bigger population than the sort of communities which appear most likely to promote consumer involvement. There is overwhelming evidence of an inverse relationship between size and citizen involvement — evidence which is international and by no means limited to health services. Thus a Swedish study has suggested that citizen involvement is greatest in densely populated communes with a population of less than 8,000 [19], while a review of the United States experience has suggested a figure of 20,000 as the outer-limit [20].

This would indicate that while it may be possible to devise a variety of ways of involving more consumers in the operations of the NHS — as an alternative or supplement to CHCs — this would be easiest at the lowest unit of service: the Health Centre or Group Practice. In other words, the highest level of interest is likely to be achieved when the scope and scale of the services concerned are most limited; as the scope and scale of the services increase, and with them the size of the population required to support them, so the problems of involvement become more difficult.

This point also indicates a fundamental flaw in what would otherwise seem to be a further policy option for making Community Health Councils more representative: directly elected members. Given the size of the NHS districts — which vary in population from 78,000 to over 500,000 — and given also the artificial nature of the administrative boundaries, it seems likely that the turn-out of voters would be derisorily small. This conclusion is reinforced by the experience of New Zealand which has been considering the abandonment of its directly elected health authorities [21]. Among the reasons given is public apathy. In the 1971 hospital board elections, only 36.2% of those eligible voted (a figure which would, admittedly, be considered moderately encouraging in the context of British local government elections), largely because a majority of seats were uncontested.

The New Zealand story is all the more cautionary since many hospital board areas have a small population: in some instance, there are fewer than 10,000 electors. The implication would seem to be that while small size may be a necessary condition for stimulating public interest, it is far from being a sufficient one. If the population is too small to support an effective or comprehensive public service, then apathy is a logical response. If there is an inverse relationship between size and interest, so equally there appears to be a direct relationship between power and interest. Absolute lack of power, it is tempting to conclude, leads to absolute apathy. And since Community Health Councils do not have even nominal power over services — in contrast to the New Zealand hospital boards — it is difficult to take the option of direct elections very seriously.

The case for multi-purpose consumer councils

So far the policy options have been discussed entirely within the framework of the National Health Service. But in practice, as shown in Chapter 4, the concerns of Community Health Councils have ranged far beyond the administrative boundaries of the NHS. Nor is this surprising. The inter-relationship of the various social services is generally recognised, and it is almost inevitable that an interest in health services will spill over into the personal social services, housing, social security payments, public transport and so on.

One option for future policy would therefore be to transform the Community Health Councils into statutory Community Consumer Councils, charged with representing consumer views in all public services — whether operated by local or central government or by public corporations. This would anticipate the possibility that the creation of CHCs may create demands for similar bodies to be set up in other public services, and so avoid the proliferation which would result if these demands were to be met. Equally, this would recognise that much consumer dissatisfaction and many consumer problems spring as much from the failure of various services to co-ordinate their activities as from the inadequacies in individual services. A National Consumer Council already exists; so why not set up similar organisations at the local level which would give the national body a constituency and the representative legitimacy which at present it so conspicuously lacks?

There is a further argument in favour of such all-purpose Community Consumer Councils: parsimony of effort and economy in the use of resources. One of the roles which many CHCs appear to be adopting informally is that of advice-giving agencies. Many people call at their offices, as seen in the last chapter, to obtain information or advice or merely to have a chat about their problems — which may or may not have anything to do with the NHS. Since there already exists a plethora of frequently under-financed advice-giving agences [22], this does not seem a particularly sensible use of public funds: it is an expensive way of advertising the existence of CHCs to the public. So while there would be a strong case for Community Consumer Councils to be financially responsible for a consolidated advice-giving service, there seems little to be said in favour of funding CHCs to develop a narrowly specialised health service information office. Indeed there is a positive case against such a development, since many people in search of advice or information do not know which particular service is relevant to their own problems or needs and thus may spend their time being shuttled from one specialised advice-giving agency to another.

In this, and in other ways as well, an all-purpose Community Consumer Council would have the advantage of cutting the costs to the citizen of seeking information, support for his case or help in dealing with his grievances. Instead of consumer representative bodies mirroring the complexity of social and other public services, they would offer a one-entry door into what is so often now a confused and perplexing world. In addition, they would be carrying out the function envisaged for the elected local councils by the Royal Commission on Local Government [23]. These councils were not to have statutory responsibility for any local services, although they would have limited powers to raise money; instead, "their key function should be to focus opinion about anything that effects the well-being of each community, and to bring it to bear on the responsible authorities". The local councils were not, in the event, set up. But there could hardly be a better definition of the main role of Community Consumer Councils.

A Community Consumer Council could not, of course, hope to acquire the depth of knowledge which a Community Health Council can expect to achieve for the more limited area of the NHS. Neither could it carry out, for the whole range of public services, the kind of information-gathering and semi-inspectorial exercises which many CHCs now perform. To settle for this option would be to settle also for a more limited model of consumer representation: one which puts the emphasis on articulating, aggregating and voicing the views of individuals and groups, as against defining interests and diagnosing problems which those affected may themselves be unable to express. Equally it would be to stress the role of proclaiming the consumer's view, as distinct from involvement in the policy or management process. So while this option has obvious attractions, the price to be paid might well be a dilution of consumer involvement in the specific circumstances of the National Health Service.

The case for local government control

In the discussion so far of the various options, much has been made about the need for legitimacy and for multi-purpose authorities. This is to invite the obvious riposte that multi-purpose authorities with unchallenged credentials to legitimacy already exist. Why re-invent the wheel, when it already exists, in the shape of local authorities? The solution to the various problems raised, it may well be argued, is to transfer control of the National Health Service to local authorities. Then, by definition, the consumer would be represented: for who is the local government elector, if not the consumer?

Taking a long view of possible policy options, this is clearly a strong runner. In principle, as pointed out in the first chapter, both the main political parties — Labour and Conservative — have accepted that such a transfer would be desirable. In practice, there are a variety of difficulties.

The present local authority boundaries were drawn up without much regard to the needs of the NHS, and frequently do not provide a satisfactory basis for building up a comprehensive health system [24]. Equally, transferring control would mean transferring financial responsibility, and it is less than clear that local authorities have the necessary capacity to raise the required revenue.

More important, in the context of the present analysis, is that consumer representation cannot be equated with control by elected councillors without very considerable qualification. At best, representing the consumer of services may be one of many roles played by councillors. But they also have a variety of others, which may well be in conflict with the function of speaking for the consumer. Like members of Hospital Management Committees, councillors may be involved in the management of particular services, and thus face the problem of divided loyalties. Equally, they may see themselves as defining some general community or public interest, which may be incompatible with the concerns of consumers in a particular service: they may, consequently, see it as their duty to explain to consumers why they cannot have what they want, instead of acting as advocates for them.

Indeed the evidence suggests that there may be a demand for some sort of institutionalised consumer voice even in services run by local authorities: after all, the interest in promoting citizen involvement first began to be expressed in the field of town planning — a local authority responsibility [25]. And the demand has been strengthened because — to take up a point made in the previous section — the logic of service provision has produced larger populations in the reorganised local authorities than might have been produced by the logic of promoting consumer involvement.

There is a further problem. It is often assumed that locally-controlled services can be equated with accessible, responsive and open services: what might be called a democratic style of administration. But while there may be strong arguments in favour of decentralisation — particularly on the grounds that government is now overloaded [26] — it cannot be taken for granted that the result would be to encourage these particular values. The little evidence that is available points in the opposite direction: it suggests that local authorities are perceived to be less responsive and less open than central government. In a survey carried out for the Commission on the Constitution [27], 73% of those interviewed agreed strongly with the statement that "The council should take more notice of the views of the people who live in the area", while only 52% agreed with the statement that "It's too difficult for ordinary people to make their views known to the government about things that affect them". And since these two statements are not identical in wording, it is worth noting — in confirmation of the pattern revealed — that while 71% of those interviewed thought that local councils do not tell people enough about what they are doing, only 63% felt the same way about central government. Similarly, 54% of those who complained to their local council offices felt that their grievances had not been dealt with satisfactorily, as against 50% of those who had complained to the civil service and 49% of those who had complained to NHS authorities.

The case for transferring control of the NHS to local authorities is therefore distinct from the case for more consumer representation. To the extent that the problems of securing accessibility, responsiveness and openness spring from the fact that the NHS is a large, complex and professionally dominated organisation — and thus inevitably tends to suffer from the pathologies which afflict such organisations — so a switch in control from central to local government would not, of itself, solve them.

The case for a national policy of accountability

This is a book about Community Health Councils, and we have therefore analysed the concept of consumer representation in the light of this particular experiment in institution-building. But, however successful, CHCs can at best be no more than one element in a complex system. To discuss them, without also taking into account the larger system of bureaucratic administration and political accountability of which they are part, is to risk exaggerating their importance and of ignoring other policy options.

The central fact about the NHS is — as already stressed — that it is a central government service, with a Secretary of State answerable to Parliament for everything that happens. Inevitably, therefore, the role of CHCs — or of any other local bodies representing the consumer — must be seen in the context of central administration and parliamentary control.

One outcome of setting up CHCs will, almost certainly, be to increase some of the stresses in the system: in particular the conflict between two competing aims of policy — the achievement of national standards and flexibility to allow local circumstances to be reflected in local services. CHCs, as we have seen, are quite ready to use national norms in order to point to deficiencies in the provision of local services; equally, however, they are quick to find reasons why special local circumstances demand extra provision for the district over and above the national norm. The same tension is evident in the relationship between local and central government, but in the case of CHCs there is not even a residual responsibility for financing extra local expenditure out of local taxation of some kind or another.

At the same time, the demands generated by what we have earlier called district patriotism are likely to be increasingly put on behalf of CHCs by members of Parliament. As it is, Parliamentary Questions and Adjournment debates are dominated by special pleading for more resources for particular localities[28], and it is clear that the creation of CHCs will reinforce this trend. There is already evidence that they are using MPs as their voice at Westminster, involving them in local campaigns for new hospitals or measures to deal with specific grievances.

So, in one respect, the in-put of information about the NHS to Parliament will increase. The creation of CHCs will have created a new channel for conveying consumer opinion to the politicians, and it may well be that the councils will be able to convey the opinions of those who are not articulate and confident enough to write to their MP off their own bat. But this will, by definition, be highly selective information sparked off by individual or community grievances. CHCs, inevitably, vary in their attitudes and in their degree of activity: some are thrusters, a few are sleepers. It cannot be taken for granted that they will necessarily be most effective in producing information about consumer views in those districts where the deficiencies in the NHS are most urgent.

So while the activities of CHCs may allow MPs to be more effective in pursuing one, limited form of accountability [29] — that which consists of calling Ministers to account for their department's actions in particular cases or particular localities — they may not contribute very much to making parliamentary control more effective in the more fundamental sense of accountability for policy decisions and policy implementations. If representing the consumer or the community is defined to mean assessing the quality of the service being provided and looking at standards — as distinct from merely voicing consumer views or grievances — then nationally Parliament is in an even weaker position than are CHCs locally.

The case for arguing that there is a wide gap between the form and substance of parliamentary accountability is familiar, and it is difficult to improve on the way it was put by the Webbs more than half a century ago [30]:

"What has happened, in fact, during the past half century, with the

169

continuous increase of the functions of government, has been the gradual establishment of a largely unselfconscious bureaucratic conspiracy against Parliamentary interference or control. The Minister, overwhelmed with the immensity of the administration for which he is nominally responsible, welcomes the assistance of his able and well-trained officials in keeping at arm's length, not only the newspapers and the public, but also the inquisitive M.P. Official secrecy becomes a disease. The evasion of questions in the House is reduced to a fine art... Discussions on the estimates are as far as possible curtailed. The happiest Ministers, and the most complacent departments, are those to which the House of Commons can be hypnotised into giving the least attention. Parliamentary control, even over policy, has become an illusion and a sham. Ministers and officials have the excuse that, as things are at present arranged, the pertinacity of Members of Parliament is almost always badly informed, the criticisms are ill-instructed, the discussions in Parliament usually extraordinarily futile; and 'Parliamentary control' seems to them to mean merely an increase of official work and anxiety, without the counterbalancing advantage of useful criticism or constructive suggestions".

In some respects, this picture is over-drawn. On specific, politically highly salient issues, Parliament can and does exercise more influence than the Webbs allow [31]. But in other respects, the conclusions have gained in strength since 1920. What the Webbs then diagnosed as the "hypertrophy of business in the House of Commons and the Cabinet" has become infinitely more acute since they wrote. The range of business demanding attention from the individual MP has widened greatly. His ability to respond, despite the provision of more secretarial and other help, has increased only modestly. And what goes for MPs individually also applies to Parliament collectively: the development of the Expenditure Committee with sub-committees specialising in particular policy-areas, has somewhat strengthened Parliament's ability to inquire into the affairs of government departments while stopping well-short of a developed capacity to scrutinise the affairs of an organisation as vast, complex and decentralised as the NHS. Dependent largely on evidence provided by the Departments, lacking any sort of investigatory staff of its own, the Expenditure Committee may be able to ask awkward questions but can seldom scrutinise the development and implementation of policy in an on-going and systematic way.

The Webbs, in considering ways of dealing with the crisis of government, put much emphasis on "the combination of measurement with publicity". Somewhat optimistically, perhaps, they concluded that "the deliberate intensification of this searchlight of published knowledge" would prove to be the "corner-stone of successful Democracy", rendering obsolete the conflicts between rulers and ruled, the administers and the administered. Not consultation but rational inquiry would, in this view, wash away conflicts. If "comparative statistics" revealed a particular service to be inadequate or wasteful, then appropriate action would follow as people were shamed into being rationally efficient.

In retrospect, this may seem a naive view. But if information about the preformance of public services does not dissolve the antagonisms of opposed interests, it is one of the ingredients in policy-making. If MPs or Community Health Councils are going to use information about the NHS then it is better — other things being equal — that they should use accurate information, rather than relying on generalisations based on individual cases or other scraps of knowledge. Hence the case for a National Health Services Audit Bureau which would carry out an on-going critical assessment of the NHS, and report annually on the state of the system to Parliament and so also to a wider audience including CHCs.

There are a number of objections to this option. The first is that there is no acceptable and accepted means of measuring or assessing the performance of the NHS. A financial audit — of the kind which the Auditor and Comptroller-General carried out on behalf of Parliament into government spending — is primarily designed to check that the money is being spent properly and, to a lesser degree, that it is being spent efficiently. Even an extended system of financial audit might be helpful in the case of the NHS, as in the case of local government. The 1976 Layfield Committee [32] recommended that the audit service for local government should be given an increased role, and encouraged to carry out studies into the efficient use of manpower. Its conclusion applies equally well to the NHS:

> "In the course of our inquiry we noted a tacit assumption by most people and organisations concerned with local authority services that, given the personalised nature of those services, particularly education and the social services, the only way to improve them is to increase manpower... We believe that even in services such as education and the social services there may well be ways of employing existing staff resources to better advantage. It would be appropriate for all services to be subjected to special study from time to time with the aim of finding ways of increasing productivity".

But, clearly, a National Health Services Audit Bureau would have to range far more widely if it were to present an analysis of the quality of the service being provided. If it were to use only the tools of accountancy, its usefulness would be limited. It would inevitably have to look at the way resources were being used, which means not only drawing on available but much under-analysed statistics, but also translating such statistics into the language of standards of care. This, in turn, would imply some sort of inspectorial system: one option might be, for example, to incorporate an extended Health Advisory Service into such an Audit Bureau.

The second main criticism of this approach is that there is already an excess of monitoring in the NHS. Not only are CHCs supposed to be assessing the service, but the work of the District Management Team is being monitored by the Area Health Authority, while the AHA is being monitored by the Regional Health Authority which, in turn, is being monitored by the Department of Health and Social Security. Everybody, in short, appears to be assessing and auditing everybody else's performance.

But this, of course, is precisely the problem: with so many layers of responsibility involved, it is far from clear what standards and criteria are being applied by whom — all the more so since the results of most of the monitoring exercises are never published. In addition, given the sheer difficulty of assessing quality and effectiveness in a health service, diffused monitoring is also likely to mean poor monitoring. The creation of a National Audit Bureau might thus make it easier to simplify the structure of the NHS by making one of the present tiers of administration even more redundant than it is already, while also making it less necessary for the DHSS to exercise control through detailed scrutiny.

To make this last point is to stress yet again that, since the present form of the National Health Service is not set in concrete for all time, the policy options for consumer representation must be seen in the context of the policy options for more fundamental changes in the system as a whole. The structure may be streamlined; boundaries may be altered; the role of central government may change. This is why we have resisted the temptation of concluding this book by making specific policy recommendations, as distinct from exploring the concept of consumer representation and various available options — a list which, in any case, cannot be exhaustive. There is no one best way of introducing consumer representation or involvement into a system such as the NHS, irrespective of the overall design of the system; different designs for the structure will inevitably demand different ways of approaching this particular problem. And while it would be perverse to suggest that any re-design of the system should revolve round the issue of consumer representation, the experience of the Community Health Councils does suggest that this consideration should be one of the elements in the discussion from the start — instead of, as in their case, being a postscript to the main debate.

1 Rudolf Klein 'Is there a case for private practice?' *British Medical Journal* 6 December 1975.

2 Rudolf Klein 'The doctors' dilemma for accountability' *Public Administration Bulletin* No.14 December 1974.

3 No such analysis is attempted, for example, in the Department of Health and Social Security's own annual review *On the State of the Public Health* (most recently issued for 1974, HMSO 1976). This looks at mortality and morbidity without relating these, for the most part, to the health services. For the difficulties of so doing, see Rudolf Klein *Social policy and public expenditure* Centre for Studies in Social Policy 1974 and *Inflation and Priorities* Centre for Studies in Social Policy 1975.

4 Rudolf Klein 'Accountability in the National Health Service' *Political Quarterly* Vol.42 No.4 Oct./Dec.1974.

5 In this, the discussion draws on Albert O. Hirschman *Exit, voice and loyalty* Harvard University Press 1970. For a discussion of how Hirschman's ideas apply to public services like health, see Dennis R. Young 'Exit and voice in the organization of public services' *Social Science Information* Vol.XIII No.3 1974. For a convincing argument that the willingness to voice grievances depends on the availability of the exit option, see A.H. Birch 'Economic models in political science: the case of exit, voice and loyalty' *British Journal of Political Science* Vol.5 No.1 January 1975.

6 Arthur Seldon *After the NHS* Institute of Economic Affairs 1968.

7 For this whole theme, see Mancur Olson *The logic of collective action Harvard University Press 1965.*

8 Rudolf Klein 'Political models and the National Health Service' in Roy M. Acheson and Lesley Air (eds.) *Seminars in Community Medicine Vol.1* Oxford University Press 1976.

9 For a highly relevant study bearing on this point, although it does not refer specifically to the NHS, see Harold L. Wilensky *Organizational Intelligence* Basic Books 1967.

10 The most interesting example in this context is France which, even more than Britain, has a tradition of administrative centralisation. See, for example, Thierry Aulagnon and Daniel Janicot 'La communication entre Administration et Administres' *La Revue Administrative* May/June 1975 and Michel Crozier *et al. Decentraliser les responsibilites — pourquoi, comment?* La Documentation Francaise 1976.

11 Rudolf Klein 'Power, democracy and the NHS' *British Medical Journal* 29 May 1976.

12 G.D.H. Cole *Guild Socialism Re-Stated* Leonard Parsons 1920. See also the author's, *Social Theory* Methuen 1920. For a contemporary comment on the implications of worker participation in the control of industry and services, see National Consumer Council *Industrial democracy and consumer democracy* NCC 1976.

13 Rudolf Klein 'A policy for change' *British Medical Journal* 7 February 1976. The consultation procedure is illustrated in Department of Health and Social Security circular *Closure or change of use of health buildings* HSC (IS)207 October 1975.

14 The ideas of the 'sixties are expounded in Department of Health and Social Security *The functions of the District General Hospital* HMSO 1969; the ideas of the 'seventies are examined in 'Nuclear hospitals' *British Medical Journal* 14 January 1976.

15 For the relationship between districts and areas, see Janet Lewis and S.

Weiner 'View from the Districts' *British Medical Journal* 5 July 1975.

16 Second Report from the Select Committee on Nationalised Industries 1970/71 *Relations with the Public* HMSO 1971 HC 514 Appendix 16, A.H. Hanson 'Principles of consumer consultation'.

17 Department of Health and Social Security circular *Appointments to Community Health Councils* HC(76)25 May 1976.

18 Department of the Environment consultation paper *Neighbourhood Councils in England* 30 July 1974.

19 Quoted in Robert A. Dahl and Edward R. Tufte *Size and democracy* Stanford University Press 1973.

20 Robert K. Yin, William A. Lucas, Peter L. Szanton and J. Andrew Spindler *Citizen organizations; increasing client control over services* Rand April 1973 R-1196-HEW.

21 Minister of Health *A Health Service for New Zealand* Government Printer 1974 H.23.

22 For an examination of this whole area, see Rosalind Brooke *Information and Advice Services* G. Bell & Sons 1972.

23 Royal Commission on Local Government in England Volume 1. *Report* HMSO 1969 Cmnd.4040.

24 M.J. Buxton and Rudolf Klein 'Distribution of Hospital Provision: policy themes and resource variations' *British Medical Journal* 6 February 1975.

25 For a general analysis, see Dilys M. Hill *Participating in Local Affairs* Penguin Books 1970. More specifically, see Committee on Public Participation in Planning *People and Planning* HMSO 1969.

26 Anthony King 'Overload: Problems of Governing in the 1970s' *Political Studies* Vol.XXIII Nos.2 to 3 June to September 1975. Also Richard Rose *Overloaded Governments* University of Strathclyde Mimeo. March 1975.

27 Commission on the Constitution Research Papers 7 *Devolution and other aspects of Government: an attitudes survey* HMSO 1973 Tables 17 and 25.

28 Rudolf Klein *The politics of health, 1948-1976* In preparation. An analysis of parliamentary questions bearing on the NHS was carried out by Dr. Renuka Rajkumar.

29 The standard work on accountability is E.L. Normanton *The accountability and audit of Governments* Manchester University Press 1966.

30 Sidney and Beatrice Webb *A Constitution for the Socialist Commonwealth of Great Britain* Longmans, Green & Co. 1920.

31 For two contrasting views about the influence of MPs, see Ronald Butt *The power of Parliament* Constable 1967 and John P. Mackintosh *The British Cabinet* (second edition) Stevens & Sons 1968. For an account of how MPs themselves view the situation, see Anthony King *British Members of Parliament: a self-portrait* Macmillan 1974.

32 *Local Government Finance: a report of the committee of inquiry* HMSO 1976. Cmnd. 6453.

Appendix A

1.A THE BALANCE OF SEXES: COMPOSITION OF CHCs BY REGIONS

The initial figure in each column is the average percentage for the region: R%. The figures in brackets give the range for the CHCs within the relevant region: Max-min.*

Region	Male R%	Male Max-min.	Female R%	Female Max-min.	% not stated	Total no. of respondents	Males in the population[1] (%)
East Anglia	50	(61 — 36)	49	(64 — 39)	1	148	49
Mersey	62	(79 — 47)	38	(53 — 21)	0	229	48
Northern	54	(67 — 39)	46	(61 — 33)	0	315	49
North East Thames	54	(71 — 35)	45	(65 — 29)	1	251	48.5
North West Thames	48	(56 — 36)	52	(64 — 44)	0	327	49
North Western	54	(89 — 44)	46	(56 — 11)	0	270	48
Oxford	58	(63 — 54)	42	(46 — 37)	0	139	47
South East Thames	50	(65 — 35)	50	(65 — 35)	0	288	48
South West Thames	48	(69 — 35)	51	(65 — 23)	1	185	47
South Western	64	(88 — 42)	36	(58 — 13)	0	230	48
Trent	55	(73 — 19)	45	(81 — 27)	0	315	49
Wales	71	(85 — 33)	28	(67 — 15)	1	364	48.5
Wessex	56	(71 — 40)	41	(60 — 29)	2	124	49
West Midlands	60	(82 — 39)	40	(61 — 18)	0	361	49.5
Yorkshire	59	(67 — 39)	41	(61 — 33)	0	250	48.5
Total:	56.5		43		0.5	3,796	49

* Thus the first figure in brackets shows the highest percentage for the appropriate category for any one CHC within the region, while the second figure shows the equivalent lowest figures. Only CHCs with a response rate of 60% and above have been included for this particular purpose.
1. Calculated from figures supplied by the DHSS.

2.A AGE DISTRIBUTION OF CHCs AND REGIONAL POPULATION[1]

	15-44 Survey %	15-44 popula-tion %	45-64 Survey %	45-64 popula-tion %	65 + Survey %	65 + popula-tion %
East Anglia	27	51	52	30	20	19
Mersey	21	52	60	31	17	17
Northern	24	51	58	31	18	17
North East Thames	33	51	53	31	14	18
North West Thames	36	53	51	30	12	16
North Western	29	50	60	31	12	19
Oxford	37	56	51	28.5	10	15.5
South East Thames	25	48	63	31	11	21
South West Thames	34	49	53	31	11	20
South Western	20	47	61	31	18	21
Trent	27	51	61	31	12	17
Wales	17	49	65	32	17	19
Wessex	21	50	60	30	16	20
West Midlands	32	53	56	31	11	16
Yorkshire	29	51	55	31	16	18
Total:	28		57		14	

1. Total population calculated from figures supplied by the DHSS.

3.A SOCIAL CLASS OF CHC MEMBERS BY REGIONS

The initial figure in each column is the average percentage for the region: R%.
The figures in brackets give the range for the CHCs within the relevant region: Max-min.*

Region	Professional and intermediate		Other non-manual		Skilled & other manual workers		% not classified	
	R%	Max-min.	R%	Max-min.	R%	Max-min.		
East Anglia	64	(89—58)	19	(22—4)	13	(22—0)	4	(N = 148)
Mersey	51	(72—35)	27	(37—11)	20	(39—10)	2	(N = 229)
Northern	51	(62—29)	27	(50—7)	18	(29—5)	5	(N = 315)
North East Thames	59	(79—53)	29	(40—15)	7	(13—0)	5	(N = 251)
North West Thames	69	(93—40)	20	(35—7)	9	(20—0)	2	(N = 327)
North Western	51	(67—32)	30	(43—17)	16	(37—5)	4	(N = 271)
Oxford	62	(79—56)	22	(33—13)	15	(12—5)	1	(N = 139)
South East Thames	54	(86—40)	27	(41—5)	6	(15—0)	14	(N = 288)
South West Thames	67	(75—53)	23	(40—8)	6	(15—0)	3	(N = 185)
South Western	56	(80—40)	27	(47—7)	10	(31—0)	6	(N = 230)
Trent	44	(73—27)	33	(52—11)	20	(58—6)	3	(N = 315)
Wales	45	(67—27)	29	(73—11)	21	(45—0)	4	(N = 364)
Wessex	62	(72—65)	27	(29—13)	9	(20—0)	2	(N = 124)
West Midlands	49	(67—35)	26	(44—17)	21	(35—0)	5	(N = 361)
Yorkshire	47	(59—27)	34	(44—19)	15	(33—0)	4	(N = 249)
Total	54		27		15		5	(N = 3,796)

* Thus the first figure in brackets shows the highest percentage for the appropriate category for any one CHC within the region, while the second figure shows the equivalent lowest figures. Only CHCs with a response rate of 60% and above have been included for this particular purpose.

180

4.A   SCHOOLS ATTENDED SINCE THE AGE OF ELEVEN

	Elementary	Comprehensive	Secondary Modern	Grammar	Public	Other	Not stated	
	%	%	%	%	%	%	%	
East Anglia	22	0	9	55	34	2	1	123% (N = 148)
Mersey	44	0	7	53	18	6	2	130% (N = 229)
Northern	40	1	12	50	19	4	1	126% (N = 315)
North East Thames	26	1	8	49	28	4	2	118% (N = 251)
North West Thames	21	1	9	48	38	4	1	122% (N = 327)
North Western	35	0	13	59	17	3	0	127% (N = 271)
Oxford	28	1	11	50	29	6	1	126% (N = 139)
South East Thames	30	1	8	50	29	8	0	126% (N = 288)
South West Thames	15	2	6	44	45	5	1	118% (N = 185)
South Western	24	0	6	43	38	4	2	117% (N = 230)
Trent	32	1	15	49	20	5	3	125% (N = 315)
Wales	49	0	10	63	10	6	1	139% (N = 364)
Wessex	31	0	4	47	35	8	3	128% (N = 124)
West Midlands	32	2	10	51	24	8	0	127% (N = 361)
Yorkshire	37	2	12	53	22	5	1	132% (N = 249)
Total:	30	1	10	51	26	5	1	124% (N = 3,796)

5.A   FULL-TIME FURTHER EDUCATION BY REGION

	No further education	University	Polytechnic	Teacher Training	Technical college/ College of Further Education	Other further education	Not stated	
	%	%	%	%	%	%	%	
East Anglia	48	26	3	10	9	3	7	106% (N = 148)
Mersey	57	19	2	8	8	3	7	104% (N = 229)
Northern	55	17	3	7	8	3	10	103% (N = 315)
North East Thames	46	31	7	5	9	2	5	105% (N = 251)
North West Thames	38	37	6	6	11	4	6	108% (N = 327)
North Western	54	21	3	8	15	1	4	106% (N = 271)
Oxford	39	29	3	9	7	7	13	107% (N = 139)
South East Thames	52	20	4	6	6	14	5	107% (N = 288)
South West Thames	40	31	7	8	9	7	8	110% (N = 185)
South Western	45	19	5	5	10	8	11	103% (N = 230)
Trent	45	18	3	9	14	4	11	104% (N = 315)
Wales	46	20	1	8	9	4	14	102% (N = 364)
Wessex	44	24	2	11	7	10	9	107% (N = 124)
West Midlands	43	25	4	6	16	6	7	107% (N = 361)
Yorkshire	46	19	4	6	16	4	11	106% (N = 249)
Total:	47	23	4	7	11	5	9	106% (N = 3,796)

6.A   MEMBERSHIP OF VOLUNTARY ORGANISATIONS BY REGIONS: SPECIAL CARE GROUPS

	Mentally handi-capped		Mental health		Physically disabled		The elderly		Children and maternity			No. of CHCs
East Anglia	22	15%	20	14%	27	18%	33	22%	21	14%	(N = 148)	7
Mersey	30	13%	26	11%	43	19%	67	29%	24	10%	(N = 229)	12
Northern	32	10%	14	4%	42	13%	75	24%	26	8%	(N = 315)	17
North East Thames	32	13%	21	8%	38	15%	67	27%	23	9%	(N = 251)	17
North West Thames	46	14%	54	17%	55	17%	72	22%	38	12%	(N = 327)	18
North Western	35	13%	20	7%	51	19%	77	29%	24	9%	(N = 271)	14
Oxford	14	10%	13	9%	24	17%	29	21%	15	11%	(N = 139)	7
South East Thames	18	6%	22	8%	39	14%	45	16%	19	7%	(N = 288)	16
South West Thames	28	15%	37	20%	27	15%	42	23%	25	14%	(N = 185)	14
South Western	33	14%	15	7%	33	14%	54	23%	21	9%	(N = 230)	14
Trent	38	12%	24	8%	53	17%	85	27%	35	11%	(N = 315)	18
Wales	45	12%	27	7%	57	16%	123	34%	29	8%	(N = 364)	22
Wessex	19	15%	16	13%	24	19%	31	25%	16	13%	(N = 124)	10
West Midlands	60	17%	37	10%	50	14%	83	23%	32	9%	(N = 361)	22
Yorkshire	38	15%	27	11%	37	15%	59	24%	23	9%	(N = 249)	17
Total Survey	490	13%	373	10%	600	16%	942	25%	371	10%	(N = 3,796)	225

The South East Thames is not included in Figure 2.5 as the results are not completely comparable with the other regions.

7.A MEMBERSHIP OF VOLUNTARY ORGANISATIONS BY REGIONS: HEALTH OR SOCIAL SERVICES

	Friends of the hospital		Organisations providing health or social services or advice		Professional organisations involved in health or social services		Any other health or social work organisation		Organisations primarily concerned with immigrants		
East Anglia	20	14%	66	45%	18	12%	18	12%	2	1%	(N = 148)
Mersey	29	13%	103	45%	21	9%	41	18%	4	2%	(N = 229)
Northern	37	12%	118	37%	30	10%	41	13%	4	1%	(N = 315)
North East Thames	47	19%	92	37%	29	12%	33	13%	25	10%	(N = 251)
North West Thames	54	17%	125	38%	45	14%	47	14%	27	8%	(N = 327)
North Western	35	13%	110	41%	37	14%	33	12%	11	4%	(N = 271)
Oxford	21	15%	42	30%	23	17%	20	14%	10	7%	(N = 139)
South East Thames	31	11%	104	36%	13	5%	29	10%	n.a.		(N = 288)
South West Thames	51	28%	69	37%	25	14%	34	18%	14	8%	(N = 185)
South Western	63	27%	83	36%	30	13%	22	10%	2	1%	(N = 230)
Trent	46	15%	129	41%	31	10%	45	14%	11	3%	(N = 315)
Wales	78	21%	138	38%	34	9%	35	10%	2	1%	(N = 364)
Wessex	42	34%	63	51%	15	12%	15	12%	3	2%	(N = 124)
West Midlands	43	12%	139	39%	51	14%	57	16%	31	9%	(N = 361)
Yorkshire	42	17%	104	42%	26	10%	41	16%	18	7%	(N = 249)
Total Survey	639	17%	1,485	39%	428	11%	511	13%	164	5%	(N = 3,796)

8.A MEMBERSHIP OF VOLUNTARY ORGANISATIONS BY REGIONS: CIVIC, COMMUNITY OR ACTION GROUPS

	Women's organisa-tions		Men's organisa-tions		Local community groups		National action groups		
East Anglia	36	24%	19	13%	43	29%	15	10%	(N = 148)
Mersey	30	13%	32	14%	54	24%	20	9%	(N = 229)
Northern	68	22%	31	10%	52	17%	21	7%	(N = 315)
North East Thames	30	12%	19	8%	70	28%	33	13%	(N = 257)
North West Thames	47	14%	21	6%	99	30%	47	14%	(N = 327)
North Western	50	19%	25	9%	55	20%	24	9%	(N = 271)
Oxford	28	20%	10	7%	35	25%	14	10%	(N = 139)
South East Thames	49	17%	10	3%	54	19%	13	5%	(N = 288)
South West Thames	27	15%	16	9%	77	42%	25	14%	(N = 185)
South Western	39	17%	39	17%	52	23%	19	8%	(N = 230)
Trent	70	22%	36	11%	70	22%	24	8%	(N = 315)
Wales	51	14%	42	12%	79	22%	20	5%	(N = 364)
Wessex	18	15%	21	17%	35	28%	16	13%	(N = 124)
West Midlands	72	20%	37	10%	94	26%	43	12%	(N = 361)
Yorkshire	30	12%	26	10%	46	18%	26	10%	(N = 249)
Total number of Individuals	645	17%	384	10%	915	24%	360	10%	(N = 3,796)

The South East Thames is not included in Figure 2.8 as the results are not completely comparable with the other regions.

9.A   RELIGIOUS AFFILIATION BY REGIONS

Consisting of: —

	Member of a church %	Established church %	Non-Conformist %	Roman Catholics %	Non-Christian religions and sects %	No denomination stated %	
East Anglia	57	41	11	3	1	1	(N = 148)
Mersey	55	32	14	8	1	0	(N = 220)
Northern	57	34	15	6	1	0	(N = 315)
North East Thames	42	25	8	7	*	1	(N = 251)
North West Thames	45	27	11	3	4	0	(N = 327)
North Western	59	34	13	11	1	0	(N = 271)
Oxford	55	36	10	7	1	1	(N = 139)
South East Thames	31	not obtained					(N = 288)
South West Thames	53	38	9	4	3	0	(N = 185)
South Western	59	40	15	3	1	0	(N = 230)
Trent	56	37	11	6	1	1	(N = 315)
Wales	69	26	37	3	*	3	(N = 364)
Wessex	63	43	14	3	2	2	(N = 124)
West Midlands	48	29	13	4	2	1	(N = 361)
Yorkshire	55	31	16	5	2	0	(N = 249)
Total:	53	30	14	5	2	1	(N = 3,796)

The South East Thames is not included in Figure 2.8 as the results are not completely comparable with the other regions.

10.A   MEMBERSHIP OF POLITICAL PARTIES BY REGIONS

Party Membership

	Member of a political party	Conservative	Labour	Liberal	Other party	Party not stated	Position holder in the party	
	%	%	%	%	%	%	%	
East Anglia	53	22	26	5	0	1	22	(N = 148)
Mersey	53	21	24	6	*	2	29	(N = 229)
Northern	51	13	34	2	0	3	27	(N = 315)
North East Thames	59	16	39	2	*	1	28	(N = 251)
North West Thames	59	22	30	5	*	2	28	(N = 327)
North Western	62	21	34	6	1	1	30	(N = 271)
Oxford	58	27	23	6	1	1	29	(N = 139)
South East Thames	59	23	30	4	0	3	39	(N = 288)
South West Thames	54	26	18	6	1	3	26	(N = 185)
South Western	47	24	13	8	0	1	22	(N = 230)
Trent	56	17	36	2	*	2	31	(N = 315)
Wales	54	7	39	4	2	2	27	(N = 364)
Wessex	52	24	18	7	1	2	27	(N = 124)
West Midlands	56	16	34	4	1	2	28	(N = 361)
Yorkshire	52	14	26	8	0	3	27	(N = 249)
Total:	55	18	30	5	1	2	28	(N = 3,796)

11.A   REGIONAL DISTRIBUTION OF LOCAL COUNCILLORS

Councillors of: —

	Currently a councillor	County Councils	County District	Metropolitan County	Metropolitan District	London Borough	GLC	Parish	
	%	%	%	%	%	%	%	%	
East Anglia	52	9	41	0	0	0	1	26	(N = 148)
Mersey	42	10	23	3	10	0	0	13	(N = 229)
Northern	43	13	25	2	7	0	0	11	(N = 315)
North East Thames	35	3	9	0	*	22	1	2	(N = 251)
North West Thames	28	3	13	0	1	11	*	5	(N = 327)
North Western	39	6	16	2	16	0	0	3	(N = 271)
Oxford	50	17	37	0	1	0	0	16	(N = 139)
South East Thames	60	5	25	0	0	13	0	6	(N = 228)
South West Thames	40	7	21	0	1	12	0	3	(N = 185)
South Western	50	12	39	0	0	0	0	26	(N = 230)
Trent	39	7	24	3	7	0	0	14	(N = 315)
Wales	53	13	34	0	1	0	0	21	(N = 364)
Wessex	50	21	31	0	1	0	0	15	(N = 124)
West Midlands	62	11	22	2	8	0	0	9	(N = 361)
Yorkshire	39	10	17	4	12	0	0	12	(N = 249)
Total:	42	10	24	1	5	4	*	12	(N = 3,796)

12.A   POSITIONS HELD

		%
School governor	2,000	53
Magistrate	493	13
Member of a consultative council of a nationalised industry	284	7
Tribunal member	348	9
Co-opted member of a local authority	535	14
Total number of positions	3,660 (N = 3,796)	

13.A QUALIFICATIONS

		%
No qualifications	797	21
University degree or above	744	20
Professional institute final exam.	476	13
H.N.C.	63	2
Teacher training certificate/Certificate of Education	336	9
GCE 'A' level/ONC/Higher School Certificate/Matriculation	1,208	32
Professional institute intermediate exam.	165	4
GCE 'O' level/School Certificate	1,241	33
SRN/other nursing qualifications	329	9
Diploma/Certificate or other qualification in social work	265	7
Full industrial apprenticeship	305	8
Secretarial diploma	298	8
Other	332	9
Not stated	188	5
	(N = 3,796)	180%

14.A THE FUNCTION OF THE CHC

The priority attached to different functions: One is the most important

	One %	Two %	Three %	Four %	Five %	Six %		Not stated (N = 3,508)
To review the standards of local services and future plans	69	13	7	5	3	3	100% (N = 3,351)	4% 157
To advise and publicise to the man in the street the facilities available	11	36	16	12	15	10	100% (N = 3,332)	5% 176
To be concerned about the way waiting lists and appointment systems are organised	11	21	22	24	6	6	100% (N = 3,327)	5% 181
To assist people to put their complaints	3	14	24	18	19	22	100% (N = 3,325)	5% 183
To be concerned about the quality of food and amenities for patients in hospitals	2	7	15	22	31	22	100% (N = 3,319)	5% 189
To ensure that the staff of the NHS have good working conditions	3	11	15	18	16	37	100% (N = 3,320)	5% 188

15.A CLASS DISTRIBUTION OF DIFFERENT AGE GROUPS

	Professional and Managerial %	White Collar %	Blue Collar %	Unclassified %	
Under 35	64	23	11	2	100% (N = 352)
35 – 54	55	28	15	2	100% (N = 1,810)
55 and over	51	27	15	7	100% (N = 1,606)

16.A GENERAL ASSESSMENT OF SERVICES BY REGION

	Good %	Adequate %	Unsatis-factory %		Not stated
East Anglia	34	54	12	100% (N = 137)	11 7% (N = 148)
Mersey	32	48	20	100% (N = 203)	26 11% (N = 229)
Northern	38	55	7	100% (N = 274)	41 13% (N = 315)
North East Thames	24	49	27	100% (N = 202)	49 20% (N = 251)
North West Thames	27	54	19	100% (N = 255)	72 22% (N = 327)
North Western	27	52	20	100% (N = 233)	37 14% (N = 270)
Oxford	30	48	22	100% (N = 115)	24 17% (N = 139)
South East Thames		Not available			
South West Thames	28	57	15	100% (N = 165)	20 11% (N = 185)
South Western	42	43	15	100% (N = 196)	34 15% (N = 230)
Trent	27	46	27	100% (N = 266)	49 16% (N = 315)
Wales	37	47	15	100% (N = 344)	20 5% (N = 364)
Wessex	38	54	7	100% (N = 114)	10 8% (N = 124)
West Midlands	28	46	26	100% (N = 322)	39 11% (N = 361)
Yorkshire	38	52	10	100% (N = 224)	26 10% (N = 250)
Total:	32	50	18	100% (N = 3,050)	458 13% (N = 3,508)

17.A   PRIORITY FOR GROUPS

The groups in the population which were considered should get priority for better services in the next few years: One is the first priority.

	One %	Two %	Three %	Four %	Five %	Six %	Seven %	Eight %		Not stated (N = 3,508)
Acutely ill patients	22	11	11	11	13	13	10	9	100% (N = 3,138)	11% 370
Elderly	20	15	13	14	13	10	8	7	100% (N = 3,141)	10% 367
Mentally handicapped	16	18	15	13	10	10	10	8	100% (N = 3,135)	11% 373
Mentally ill	16	19	17	15	11	10	8	4	100% (N = 3,137)	11% 371
Ordinary patients	12	9	7	9	12	11	13	27	100% (N = 3,132)	11% 376
Physically handicapped	6	13	17	19	16	15	10	4	100% (N = 3,130)	11% 378
Children	6	10	12	13	16	19	17	5	100% (N = 3,126)	11% 382
Maternity	2	6	7	7	8	12	23	35	100% (N = 3,122)	11% 386

18.A   REGIONAL DIFFERENCES IN THE PRIORITIES GIVEN TO PARTICULAR GROUPS

		Acutely ill patients	Elderly	Mentally handicapped	Mentally ill	Ordinary patients	Physically handicapped	Children	Maternity
East Anglia	First priority	20%	23%	13%	20%	14%	5%	4%	2%
	Mean rank	4.11	3.86	4.16	3.50	4.62	4.35	4.92	6.44
Mersey	First priority	29%	16%	10%	19%	13%	7%	6%	1%
	Mean rank	3.59	4.06	4.35	4.20	5.37	4.13	4.46	6.16
Northern	First priority	24%	20%	19%	13%	10%	8%	5%	1%
	Mean rank	4.05	3.75	3.82	3.59	5.35	4.20	4.80	6.31
North East Thames	First priority	16%	19%	16%	22%	16%	3%	6%	2%
	Mean rank	4.40	3.91	3.83	3.30	5.12	4.51	4.79	5.90
North West Thames	First priority	12%	20%	22%	25%	7%	8%	5%	1%
	Mean rank	4.85	3.69	3.32	2.96	5.72	4.05	4.94	6.37
North Western	First priority	25%	16%	14%	14%	14%	6%	11%	2%
	Mean rank	3.90	3.80	4.23	3.91	5.01	4.39	4.47	6.16
Oxford	First priority	23%	26%	13%	18%	14%	5%	2%	0%
	Mean rank	4.00	3.61	4.13	3.53	5.10	4.24	5.13	6.13
South West Thames	First priority	14%	24%	15%	22%	13%	9%	7%	0%
	Mean rank	4.66	3.58	3.87	3.32	4.86	4.09	5.01	6.38
South Western	First priority	18%	24%	19%	14%	14%	8%	3%	2%
	Mean rank	4.05	3.61	3.78	3.84	4.92	4.25	5.10	6.28
Trent	First priority	26%	14%	15%	12%	15%	7%	11%	2%
	Mean rank	3.78	4.20	4.09	3.98	5.14	4.36	4.35	5.99
Wales	First priority	30%	24%	15%	10%	9%	5%	6%	1%
	Mean rank	3.66	3.52	3.91	4.11	5.20	4.25	4.76	6.27
Wessex	First priority	21%	23%	18%	12%	8%	5%	10%	3%
	Mean rank	4.11	3.86	3.99	3.94	5.28	4.31	4.78	5.72
West Midlands	First priority	26%	16%	15%	14%	12%	6%	9%	3%
	Mean rank	3.68	4.22	4.07	3.85	4.98	4.57	4.39	6.02
Yorkshire	First priority	20%	27%	18%	16%	9%	6%	4%	2%
	Mean rank	4.23	3.58	3.50	3.55	5.73	4.09	4.96	6.20

Appendix B - Survey methods

Community Health Councils were set up over a period of time, and the long delays in completing the process meant that our postal survey had to be carried out on the instalment plan. The South East Thames and Wessex regions had both set up most of their CHCs by the end of April 1974 — the target-day set by the Department of Health and Social Security — and it was agreed that our pilot survey should be carried out in the former. This was done, and our questionnaire was amended in the light of the experience gained there: it is printed in its final form at the end of this appendix. Meanwhile, more regions had set up their CHCs and in the autumn of 1974 questionnaires were sent out to members in 12 regions. The survey, like the process of setting up CHCs, was completed in 1975 when first the Welsh and then the West Midlands members were sent their questionnaires: at the beginning of the year and in June, respectively.

In the pilot region, the South East Thames, the questionnaires were distributed on our behalf by the CHC secretaries to the individual members who mailed the replies back to us. For the main survey, a different method was used: the names and addresses of all CHC members were obtained from the regional authorities, and questionnaires were mailed direct to them. One reminder was sent to non-respondents. Previously, steps had been taken to make the CHC members aware of the survey, to introduce them to the aims of the study and to re-assure them that the Centre for Studies in Social Policy was an independent institute with no axe to grind. The best way of doing so was discussed with the regional administrators, and slightly different approaches were adopted in different regions. In four of them, the regional administrator or his colleague mentioned our survey at the inaugural meetings of CHCs; in four others we sent a preliminary letter to all CHC chairmen; in Wales, the Welsh Office wrote to CHC chairmen enclosing a letter from the Centre and in the remaining five regions no formal introductions were made and a questionnaire was sent direct to CHC members.

The survey encountered some resistance. Some CHCs formally debated whether or not their members should fill in the questionnaire, and four in the North Western region opted out of the survey altogether. In one case, too, the regional chairman strongly expressed his suspicion of all surveys and was only persuaded with some difficulty not to excommunicate ours. Additional difficulties were encountered in the South East Thames and Wessex region where, without advance consultation, the Office of Health Economics sent out a questionnaire to CHC members shortly before ours. This duplication unfortunately produced some antagonism to surveys and probably affected the response rate in these two regions.

Even so, the overall response rate was 64.7%, as shown in Table 1B which also gives the regional break-down for the number of questionnaires sent out. The response rate is, strictly speaking, not a percentage of all CHC members but only of those who were in office at the time the surveys were carried out. Some had not yet been appointed. Others had resigned. A few had died. As far as the available information allows, allowance has been made for all these factors. No attempt was made to update the information by sending questionnaires to councillors who were appointed after the survey was well under way.

There were considerable variations both between regions and individual councils in the proportion of members replying to the questionnaire. The distribution of these response rates is given in Table 2B. There do not appear to be any systematic patterns in the differences of response and we have therefore assumed that the variations are random. Lacking an independent data base for CHC councillors, we can only test our sample for bias in one respect. Given the method of nominating CHC members, the distribution for the various nominating bodies ought to be 50% for local authority nominees, 33% for voluntary organisation nominees and 17% for RHA nominees. In fact, of the respondents in our survey 46% were local authority nominees, 38% were voluntary organisation nominees and 16% were RHA nominees. This would suggest that voluntary organisation members were over-represented, and local authority members were under-represented. However, this could be a function less of response bias than of the fact that some local authorities were rather slow in appointing their nominees and that, at the time of our survey, their complement had not yet been filled.

Questionnaires were returned to the Centre, and were then checked and coded by Social Policy Research Ltd., who were also responsible for card punching. Social class was classified according to the Census definitions; occupations on the basis of a list compiled at the Centre. Position held in voluntary organisations were defined in terms of election or appointment: chairman or secretary are clearly "positions" but we also put into this category those chosen by his or her organisation to represent it on another body, such as the Council for Social Service. The computing of the data was carried out by Alan Joy at London University Computing Services Ltd.

1.B   RESPONSE RATES

	Number of question-naires sent out	Number of known resignations and member-ship changes	Total question-naires in survey	Total completed returns	Response rate %
East Anglia	213	—	213	148	69.5
Mersey	357	—	357	229	64.1
Northern	469	—	469	315	67.2
North East Thames	426	1	425	251	59.1
North West Thames	481	7	474	327	69.0
North Western	404	3	401	271	67.6
Oxford	203	1	202	139	68.8
South East Thames	446	—	446	288	64.6
South West Thames	317	5	312	185	59.3
South Western	325	4	321	230	71.7
Trent	473	4	469	315	67.2
Wales	541	—	541	364	67.3
Wessex	213	2	211	124	58.8
West Midlands	610	8	602	362	60.1
Yorkshire	429	2	427	249	58.3
Total:	5,907	37	5,870	3,796	64.7

2.B DISTRIBUTION OF RESPONSE RATE BY REGIONS: NUMBER OF CHCs WITHIN EACH CATEGORY

% Response rate	Under 39	40—49	50—59	60—69	70—79	80—89	90+	Total number of CHCs
East Anglia		1	1	1	3		1	7
Mersey		1	2	5	3	1		12
Northern			5	5	5	2		17
North East Thames	3		4	6	3	1		17
North West Thames		1	2	7	3	4	1	18
North Western		1	2	5	4	2		14
Oxford			2	2	1	2		7
South East Thames	1	1	4	4	5		1	16
South West Thames		4	1	6	2	1		14
South Western			2	5	3	4		14
Trent	2		1	7	4	2	2	18
Wales		2	3	5	7	5		22
Wessex	2		3	2	2	1		10
West Midlands	1	1	8	8	3	1		22
Yorkshire	3	1	5	3	4	1		17
Total:	12	13	45	71	52	27	5	225

The Questionnaire

Centre for Studies in Social Policy

62 Doughty Street London WC1N 2LS
Telephone 01-242-7236

COMMUNITY HEALTH COUNCILS SURVEY

OFFICE USE ONLY

(1)-(4)	5013

SERIAL NO:

(5)(6)(7)(8)

CHC:

(9)(10)(11)

RHA:

(12)(13)

STRICTLY CONFIDENTIAL

For each question please indicate the answer (or answers) by ticking the corresponding box e.g. [✓] or by writing in the answer.

Name of Community Health Council:

Are you the Chairman or Vice-Chairman?   (14)

Chairman	1
Vice-Chairman	2

1a Do you live in the district covered by your Community Health Council: (15)

Yes	1
No	2

1b IF YES: How long have you lived in the district?

Please write your answer in the boxes with one figure only in each box.

(16)(17)

e.g. 5 years: [0][5]

2. Which of these bodies appointed you to be a member of the Community Health Council? Please write in the name of the authority or organisation.   (18)

Local Authority	1
Voluntary Organisation	2
Regional Health Authority	3

- 2 -

3. What was your age last birthday?   OOO (19)

Under 25	1
25 - 34	2
35 - 44	3
45 - 54	4
55 - 64	5
65 and over	6

4. Are you ....   (20)

Male	1
Female	2

5. Are you ....   (21)

Married	1
Single	2
Widowed/Divorced/Separated	3

6. Do you have any children under 16 years of age? If so, how many?   (22)

None	1
One	2
Two	3
Three	4
Four	5
Five or more	6

7. What schools have you attended since the age of 11? Please tick all that apply, and write in any others not listed.   (23)

Elementary	1
Comprehensive	2
Secondary Modern	3
Grammar/Technical School	4
Public School/Private School	5
Others :	6

- 3 -

OUO

8. Please tick any of the further education establishments you have attended full-time, and write in any others not listed which you have attended full-time.

(24)

No full-time further education	1
University	2
Polytechnic/CAT	3
Teacher Training College/College of Education	4
Technical College/College of Further Education	5
Others:	6

9. Please tick any of the following qualifications which you have and write in any others you have which are not listed here.

(25)

No formal qualifications/None of these	1
University degree or above	2
Professional institute final exam	3
HNC	4
Teacher Training Certificate/Certificate of Education	5
GCE 'A' Level/ONC/Higher School Certificate/Matriculation	6
Professional Institute intermediate exam	7
GCE 'O' Level/School Certificate	8
	(26)
SRN/Other nursing qualifications	1
Diploma/Certificate or other qualification in social work	2
Full industrial apprenticeship	3
Secretarial diploma	4
Others:	

- 4 -

OUO

10. Please indicate your employment situation

(27)

Working full-time (over 30 hours a week)	1
Working part-time (8-30 hours a week)	2
Working in an unpaid capacity (over 8 hours a week)	3
A full-time housewife	4
Retired	5
Not in employment	6

11. What is your occupation? (If you are retired, a full-time housewife or not currently in paid employment, please state your main occupation whilst employed.)

OCCUPATION:

YOUR TITLE/RANK/GRADE: (28)

TYPE OF INDUSTRY/BUSINESS: (29)

Are you self-employed?   Yes   No

12a Approximately how many people are employed at the place where you work? (If you are retired, a full-time housewife or not currently in paid employment, please state the number of employees at your main place of work whilst employed.)

Less than 25 people

25 or more people

Don't know

12b For how many of these employees are you responsible?

Please write number here:

201

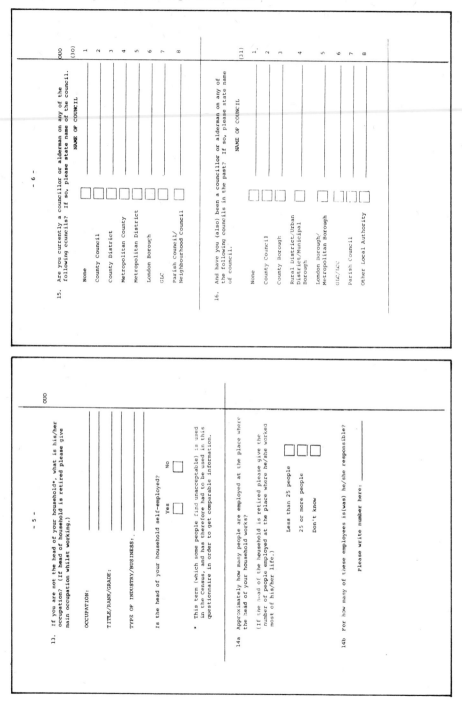

- 6 -

OOO
(30)

15. Are you currently a councillor or alderman on any of the following councils? If so, please state name of the council.

NAME OF COUNCIL

None	1
County Council	2
County District	3
Metropolitan County	4
Metropolitan District	5
London Borough	6
GLC	7
Parish Council/ Neighbourhood Council	8

(31)

16. And have you (also) been a councillor or alderman on any of the following councils in the past? If so, please state name of council.

NAME OF COUNCIL

None	1
County Council	2
County Borough	3
Rural District/Urban District/Municipal Borough	4
London Borough/ Metropolitan Borough	5
GLC/LCC	6
Parish Council	7
Other Local Authority	8

- 5 -

OOO

13. If you are not the head of your household*, what is his/her occupation? (If head of household is retired please give main occupation whilst working.)

OCCUPATION: _____

TITLE/RANK/GRADE: _____

TYPE OF INDUSTRY/BUSINESS: _____

Is the head of your household self-employed?

Yes ☐   No ☐

* This term (which some people find unacceptable) is used in the Census, and has therefore had to be used in this questionnaire in order to get comparable information.

14a Approximately how many people are employed at the place where the head of your household works?

(If the head of the household is retired please give the number of people employed at the place where he/she worked most of his/her life.)

Less than 25 people ☐
25 or more people ☐
Don't know ☐

14b For how many of these employees is(was) he/she responsible?

Please write number here: _____

- 8 -

19. Community Health Councils are supposed to represent a wide range of groups within the community. Are you a member of any of the following?

Please write the name(s) of the organisation(s) and any position(s) you hold in the one most appropriate category in each case.

HEALTH AND SOCIAL WORK ORGANISATIONS

Organisations concerned primarily with:

(38)
a) The mentally handicapped (including mentally handicapped children)
Yes ☐ 1   No ☐ 2
Organisations: _____ 3
Positions: _____

b) Mental health (39)
Yes ☐ 1   No ☐ 2
Organisations: _____ 3
Positions: _____

c) The physically disabled (40)
Yes ☐ 1   No ☐ 2
Organisations: _____ 3
Positions: _____

d) The elderly (41)
Yes ☐ 1   No ☐ 2
Organisations: _____ 3
Positions: _____

e) Children and maternity (42)
Yes ☐ 1   No ☐ 2
Organisations: _____ 3
Positions: _____

Friends of the Hospital (43)
Yes ☐ 1   No ☐ 2
Organisations: _____ 3
Positions: _____

Organisations providing health or social services and advice (including the Red Cross, St. Johns, WRVS, FPA, Councils of Social Service, CAB, Marriage Guidance etc.) (44)
Yes ☐ 1   No ☐ 2
Organisations: _____ 3
Positions: _____

- 7 -

17. Do you now, or did you in the past, hold any of the following positions? Please tick yes or no.

DO/DID YOU HOLD THIS POSITION
Yes   No   (12)
Magistrate ☐ 1   ☐ 2

School Governor or Manager (13)
Yes ☐ 1   No ☐ 2

Member of Consultative Council of a nationalised industry. PLEASE GIVE NAME OF INDUSTRY: (34)
Yes ☐ 1   No ☐ 2

Tribunal Member. PLEASE GIVE NAME OF TRIBUNAL: (35)
Yes ☐ 1   No ☐ 2

Co-opted Member of a Local Authority Committee. PLEASE GIVE NAME OF COMMITTEE AND L.A.: (36)
Yes ☐ 1   No ☐ 2

18. Have you been a member of any of the following health committees? (37)
☐☐☐☐☐☐☐☐
None   1
Hospital Management Committee   2
Regional Hospital Board   3
Local Authority Health Committee   4
Executive Council   5
Teaching Hospital Management Body   6
Hospital House Committee   7
Any other similar Committee: PLEASE GIVE NAME OF COMMITTEE BELOW: 8

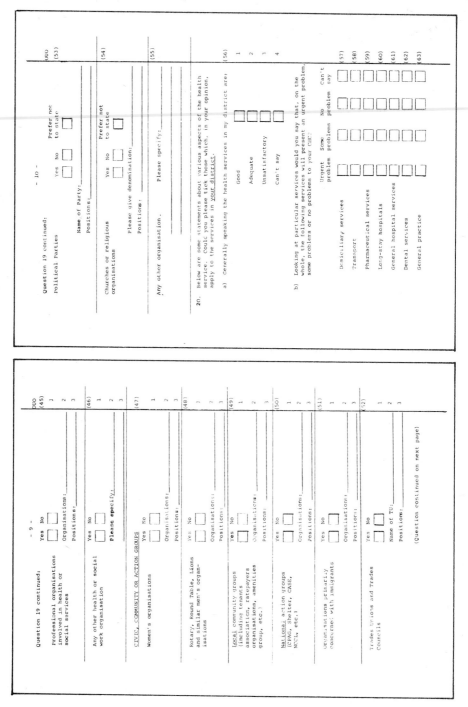

- 11 -

21. What groups in the population do you think should get priority for better services in the next few years?

   Please number in order of importance the groups listed below (i.e. put a (1) in the box by what you consider to be the group which should have first priority, a (2) against the next one in your order of priority, and so on).

   Please put a number against all of them, using the full 1 to 8 range, without ties.

Mentally handicapped	(64)
Ordinary patients	(65)
Mentally ill	(66)
Acutely ill patients	(67)
Physically handicapped	(68)
Children	(69)
Maternity cases	(70)
The elderly	(71)

22. Community Health Councils have a number of different jobs to do. Below is a list of three suggestions that have been made about their roles.

   Please rank them in order of the importance you attach to them (i.e. put a (1) in the box by what you consider the most important role, and so on).

The CHCs are essentially a channel through which the health authorities and the public can learn of each other's needs and difficulties.	(72)
The CHC's job is to represent the community's interests in the health service to those responsible for the management.	(73)
The CHC's job is to create understanding among consumers of the problems of the NHS and its staff.	(74)

- 12 -

23. Please rank the following six statements about the work of Community Health Councils in order of the importance you attach to them.

   (Again, please put a (1) in the box next to the one you consider most important, and so on, and use all 6 numbers without ties.)

   The function of the CHC is:-

to be concerned about the way waiting lists and appointment systems are organised	(75)
to be concerned about the quality of food and amenities for patients in hospitals	(76)
to review the standards of local services and future plans	(77)
to advise and publicise to the man in the street the facilities available	(78)
to assist people to put their complaints	(79)
to ensure that the staff of the NHS have good working conditions	(80)

THANK YOU FOR YOUR HELP

The Centre for Studies in Social Policy
62 Doughty Street, London, WC1N 2LS

The Centre, which is both independent and non-partisan, aims to promote the analysis and discussion of the social dimension of public policy. It provides a neutral forum where all those involved or interested in the policy process — officials, politicians, academics and others — can meet to discuss social issues. And its staff is engaged in developing the policy analysis of such issues: in particular, the Centre is concerned to examine the long-term implications of existing policies and to identify problems and policy options which are not yet on the political agenda. Its activities therefore combine the organisation of conferences and seminars and the publication of papers based on the ongoing work at the Centre.

Wherever possible, the Centre ignores conventional boundaries, whether administrative or academic. It seeks to look at social issues across departmental boundaries and across academic disciplines — and to identify the social implications of issues which are often regarded as outside the scope of social policy analysis.

The Centre was incorporated late in 1972 through the initiative and generosity of the Joseph Rowntree Memorial Trustees. It is governed by a Council of Management — listed below — drawn from a wide range of governmental, business and academic life.